The HeadWay to Health

The HeadWay to Health

Robert Boyd, D.O.

FIRST EDITION

Copyright © 1992 by Robert Boyd, D.O.

Published by Vantage Press, Inc.
516 West 34th Street, New York, New York 10001

Manufactured in the United States of America
ISBN: 0-533-10123-9

Library of Congress Catalog Card No. : 91-91421

0 9 8 7 6 5 4 3 2 1

SECOND EDITION

Copyright © 2003 by Robert Boyd, D.O.

Published by the Bio Cranial Institute, Inc.
43-44 Kissena Blvd., Flushing, New York 11355

0 9 8 7 6 5 4 3 2 1

Dedication

To James and Matthew

Contents

Foreword
by
David L. Driscoll, D.C.

It seems that within one's lifetime there are very few special people that prove to have major, significant impact. In my brief existence, Dr. Robert Boyd has been one of those select few.

Dr. Boyd has provided me the next building block in my continuing education toward a better understanding of the true definition of health. He has been more than just a teacher. He has been my mentor.

Dr. Boyd possesses a unique combination of questioning, exploration, investigation, experience, and clinical expertise. He brings to his chosen advocation of teaching unequaled enthusiasm and humor. He has a definite aptitude for the clear expression of his benchmark concepts and ideas. Dr. Boyd's passion for knowledge and his willingness and ability to share his expertise are reasons behind his special propensity for increasing the dedication and excellence of his students.

As the reader will find in this book, Dr. Boyd has illuminated the shortcomings within the philosophy and teachings of modern medicine. However, he does not leave us without an alternative. Dr. Boyd expounds possible answers to tough questions.

With the advent of chiropractic and osteopathy, a new focus on health was formed. The idealism behind both of these professions was originally the true concept of holism, or holistic healing; that is, the idea that each body is one single, whole unit and anything that affects any part of that body will impact the whole body.

Unfortunately, health care in all aspects has evolved away from this concept, including, in general, the professions of chiropractic and osteopathy.

Dr. Boyd brings us back on focus. He gives you, the reader, an elementary, pure look at the true cause of disease, or lack of optimal health. He then provides an introduction to Bio Cranial Therapy, our best chance at allowing our bodies to function as originally designed.

David L. Driscoll, D.C.
Colorado Springs, Colorado

Preface To Second Edition

In modern Western society we are assailed almost daily with stories of the latest miracles of medical science, of the promises of some new wonder drug and of the new dawn that is about to burst upon us as we explore ever deeper into the mysteries of our genetic makeup. Wonderful indeed, perhaps even frightening.

Meantime, whatever happened to the notion of *vis medicatrix naturae*, the healing power of nature? Have we forever lost sight of the essential and inherent ability of the body to *heal itself*? If the body is not able to heal itself, has it occurred to us that *there must be a reason* - or reasons? After all, are we not perfectly made? Or potentially so? Are we not endowed with the most wonderful and potentially perfect system of checks and balances to allow us to *function* at all levels of our "beingness"? Yet few of us can claim to be as near perfect as we would like to be.

So, are we as perfect as we can, or should, be? For if we were, we should surely be enjoying a high level of wellbeing. And if not, why not? Is it really possible to be functioning at a better, and more wholesome, level? Or is it just a pipe dream? " I have always been this way, so I guess it's just the way I am." The truth is that few of us have a yardstick to measure our sense of wellbeing by, for the simple reason that none of us has known, from birth, what it is like to function at our fullest potential. Function? Yes, function. For it is to a little known mechanism that we must turn to learn why we are deficient in this primary area, an area unknown to medical science and, indeed, to most healthcare professionals.

This book is an attempt to convey an important message to the reader. It is, firstly, that there is a huge untapped potential within each of us to correct much that is wrong with our health. The nature of that potential is what I have spent most of my professional life uncovering and determining how it needs to be addressed in just about every one of us.

In these pages the reader will discover that, at the very core of the myriad of functions for which - down to the activities at the very cell level itself - there exists a mechanism upon which practically every other activity depends, *and that mechanism is compromised in all of us in some degree, often to a major degree. The original name given to this approach to healthcare was Bio Cranial Therapy.® This name has now been changed to the Bio Cranial System to more accurately reflect the totality of the understandings behind this discipline. The term, Bio Cranial Therapy (BCT),® continues to be used to describe the practical work itself.*

The world of medicine, and medical men and women, is full of despair. There is no reason why it should not be full of hope and optimism.

Acknowledgments

The author gratefully acknowledges the help he has received from many sources in the compiling of this book. Special mention is here made of two of my teachers, A. W. Priest, D.O., F.N.I.M.H., of London, England, and the late Denis Brookes, Ph.D., D.O., both of whom exercised profound influences on my understanding of the health and disease processes.

My thanks also to David G. Boal, B.A., M.S., for his most valuable and constructive suggestions to improve the text and flow of ideas, and to David Driscoll, D.C., for his excellent contribution to the factual accuracy of parts of the text; and to Mrs. Linda Montgomery from my hometown of Bangor, to whom I am indebted for her help in producing most of the illustrations.

I also wish to thank Harper Collins Publishers, 77–85 Fulham Palace Road, London W6 8JB, England, for their kind permission to reprint photographs from the book *Lectures on Cranial Osteopathy*, by Denis Brookes, D.O.

I wish to express my thanks, also, to those patients who freely cooperated in agreeing to have their photographs published in this book.

The HeadWay to Health

Chapter 1

Introduction

The search for health has been one of Man's unremitting preoccupations from the beginning of time. Ill health or disease, like the poor, has always been with us. Indeed, so persistent is ill health in one form or another that it is easy to become disillusioned. In Western society we seem to be pouring massive resources into systems of health care without commensurate increases in the health of the individual.

I believe that the world of health provision has been transformed progressively into self-perpetuating empires for economic gain and professional power in which the interests of the patient are ever more subservient to these aims. But, even worse, it becomes increasingly apparent that there is a very low level of real understanding in the health care "establishment" about the very nature of the health and disease processes. All too frequently superficial and inadequate explanations are offered to sufferers of a whole range of common maladies. The purpose of this book is not to hound the empire builders of health care. Much more important, I believe, is the task of understanding the functioning of the whole human organism. If we succeed in doing so, then the means of treatment for disease become clear and the pursuit of health is greatly advanced. To illustrate how little understanding is applied in the conventional forms of medical treatment, let us consider two of the commonest reasons for a visit to the doctor: the "virus" and the "bad back."

1

The Virus

What causes ill health in the first place? The primary culprit these days seems to be the virus. Our friend—or is it enemy?—the virus has, of course, been around for a long time and with the advancing technology at our disposal we have added in recent years enormously to our knowledge of the microcosm of cellular activity. This knowledge has brought with it an awareness that in the presence of many disease, or ill-health, situations, we find aberrant viral activity. One of the unresolved questions that arises here is whether the viruses, which are often undoubtedly present, are the cause of the malady or whether they are a part of cellular change *as a result of* other and more profound disturbances within the system.

Whichever of these considerations is true—or, indeed, if either is true—there have been, from a practical point of view, two major consequences to the approach of Western medicine to a range of common and not-so-common illnesses. The first of these is that therapy has become almost entirely based upon the idea that if a virus is the "cause" of the disorder, then it has to be killed off or neutralized or modified in some way; and, in practice, this opens the field for the whole range of antibacterial and antiviral drugs, such as the antibiotics.

The second consequence is that a range of maladies, which often have rather vague and unspecific symptoms, are increasingly diagnosed as being of viral origin and are being treated with either antibiotic-type preparations or nothing at all. It is worth noting here that in these cases there is only a presumption of the presence of viral activity, which means, of course, that the diagnosis is even more unspecific. The resultant therapeutic procedures are then as much guesswork as the diagnosis. It is a rare physician who will admit that he does not know what the cause of the malady is and that drug therapy would therefore be inappropriate. The euphoric days of the discovery and introduction of the antibiotics have long since gone, but the underlying belief that bacteria and viruses are *the* cause of such a wide range of illnesses persists. The questioning of the underlying causative mechanisms and the role of bacteria/viruses as cause *or* effect has not even begun.

All this continues in spite of the observable evidence that treatment of so-called viral types of illness along orthodox lines most often results in (a) no change, (b) some diminution of symptoms temporarily, or (c) the suppression of one group of symptoms only to be replaced in a short time by another group of symptoms. In one survey, antibiotic treatment of otitis media (middle ear infection) was compared among different countries. It found that recovery did not depend on the type or duration of antibiotic treatment, and recovery rates were *higher* in those not given any antibiotic.

The viral or bacterial-based illnesses range from the well-known children's ailments such as measles and chicken pox through many common and often serious complaints such as colitis, cystitis, pleurisy, and osteomyelitis up to such a life-threatening illness as AIDS with its presumed HIV viral causation. There are schools of thought that illnesses such as certain cancers and multiple sclerosis, among others, may also have a viral origin. The word *infection* becomes synonymous with conditions which are considered to be bacterial or viral in origin. These will include such phenomena as postoperative failures to heal and suppurative processes.

In short, the view that a major range of diseases has simple bacterial or viral causes has become the sheet anchor of much of medicine's attitude to therapy. By any standards, this theory of disease is at best inadequate; at worst it is potentially dangerous.

The "Bad Back"

Musculoskeletal disorders—or to give them their more expanded title, neuromusculoskeletal (NMS) disorders—are arguably the biggest single range of illnesses handled by the family physician today. They include a wide range of painful and incapacitating conditions such as low back pain, sciatica, shoulder and arm pain, neck pain, so-called tennis elbow, and a variety of similar conditions of the extremities such as wrists, fingers, ankles, knees, and hips. What hope, then, does medicine offer this group of patients, often much maligned as exaggerating their suffering or incapacity and, indeed, frequently suspected of being malingerers?

Sadly, the answer has to be very little. The most common prescription in the first instance for many of these conditions is—not surprisingly—drug therapy. Probably the most common drugs used in such cases are straightforward analgesics or painkillers, sometimes purchased over the counter by the patient or, more likely, by prescription from the family physician. Now, on the basis that many of these conditions are both very painful and/or occur suddenly, there is no inherent objection to resorting to the use of analgesics, *providing it is looked upon as a stopgap* or an any port-in-a-storm measure. The real objection arises when it is realized that many doctors regard the prescribing of such drugs as an end to the therapy *unless* there is pressure from the patient for further investigation.

Such pressure is most likely to arise either because the pain persists or the degree of incapacity—including its domestic, business, and financial consequences—remains intolerable; at which point, the patient is likely to find himself referred for further investigation. He then enters the rather awesome and often depersonalized world of low-tech investigative medicine. A typical procedure might be as follows.

First, a consultation and examination with a consultant physician in orthopedics, who will probably indicate the need for radiological (X-ray) investigation. Having excluded the presence of any serious abnormality, which is nearly always the case, the patient is then advised: (a) that the X rays are clear (often with an implication that the problem is a figment of the patient's imagination), (b) that there is some abnormality about the alignment of some bone(s), (c) that there is some arthritis present, or (d) that there is a degeneration of a disk. At this point there is often no promising prognosis and the patient is advised that little can be done and he must learn to live with it or that some physiotherapy might help.

Either the patient gives up here or he goes to physiotherapy or, if things are sufficiently bad, he persists. If he persists, he might then go on to the high-tech stage and have further investigations such as CAT scans. It might even be decided to proceed with investigative surgery.

The message that finally begins to dawn on the more perceptive of sufferers is that no one appears to have any real understanding of the mechanisms that have gone wrong. There is often a lingering suspicion that some of the explanations were simplistic, but it is difficult to challenge the professional. The patient might think, but will rarely say, "How come, if there is arthritis in my spine, that this excruciating pain only arose when I picked up the bucket of water? After all, the arthritis must have been there for some time."

Many sufferers, though, never make such judgments, let alone express them. Instead, they become inured to a long course of drug treatment. Although analgesics are probably the most common form of prescribed drug for pain, they are not the only ones. Another group of drugs in common use nowadays are the anti-inflammatory ones such as phenylbutazone and ibuprofen, which one finds prescribed when there appears to be acute muscular spasm with some accompanying degree of inflammation. And again, resort may be made to procedures such as steroid injections where there appears to be evidence of joint inflammation, not only in diseases such as rheumatoid arthritis, but also where there is evidence of capsular inflammation, as in the frozen shoulder or tennis elbow syndromes.

Notice that all such treatment is entirely symptomatic; that is to say, the intention is merely to alleviate the symptoms with little pretense at attempting to understand and correct any more fundamental causes of the condition. We shall return to this matter later.

In this chapter I have introduced two areas of the health care issue in order to consider, briefly, the current approach to those categories of illness which fall within each. Together they constitute a major proportion of the time, effort, and money expended in the health care systems. Treatment of the first group—the viral/bacterial-based illnesses—I believe to be based on a false and inadequate understanding of cellular activity and function. Treatment of the second is based on a poor understanding of what might be called the body's mechanical function, although, as we shall see, these two gaps in understanding are not so far removed from one another as we might think. There must therefore be other questions to be asked—and, hopefully, answered.

Chapter 2

The Immune System and Germs

And lo, it came to pass that out of the heavens a swarm of germs
   descended upon the earth.
And their leader had the task of deciding where to launch their
   attack.
And it came about that he decided they would land in the colony
   of Hong Kong.
And in tribute to this, their ravages came to be known as Hong
   Kong flu.
And after twenty days and twenty nights, it was carried worldwide.
And the leader of this army was hailed as a warrior among
   warriors.
And they multiplied.
And when destruction was complete, the leader led his army back
   to the heavens whence they came.

Poor wee germ. If it isn't the virus, then it's the germ who gets
the blame for almost everything these days. But to what extent
is he the rascal? Most of us believe implicitly that Western
medicine has made enormous strides in recent years, and
particularly in the treatment of the so-called infectious and
contagious illnesses.

It has long been recognized that there is a relationship
between various illnesses such as cholera, smallpox, diph-
theria, influenza, common colds, bronchitis, measles, and the
presence within the body of some microorganism. The
originator of the modern-day germ theory, as we know it, is
generally believed to be the French chemist Louis Pasteur
(1822–95). Among other things, Pasteur laid claim to the

7

discovery of the nature of fermentation, but in fact he plagiarized the work of his contemporaries, particularly that of Professor Pierre Jacques Antoine Béchamp, one of France's greatest scientists. Béchamp was the first to demonstrate that the molds that accompanied the fermentation processes either were themselves, or contained, living organisms. They could not be spontaneously generated but had to be an outgrowth of a living organism, which could be carried in the air.

The fermentation process was then found by Béchamp to be caused by other "little bodies" within the cell which he called "microzymas," from the Greek word meaning "small ferment." After much painstaking research, he found that his microzymas, rather than the cell, were the basic units of life. He concluded then that all living organisms, from the one-cell amoeba up to Man himself, were associations of these microzymas. He described how bacteria, which others had regarded as a different species, can develop from the microzyma by passing through a number of intermediate stages. The germs of the air were merely microzymas, or bacteria, set free when their normal environment was changed.

The bacteria are therefore a mutation from a normal healthy cell which, for reasons unknown or not understood, has been disturbed to the point of being unable to maintain that level of equilibrium required for normal healthy activity. The bacteria therefore exist in the first instance and only become aberrant in behavior when the normality of cellular environment is upset. This metamorphosis from what Béchamp called a microzyma to a bacterium must be an intelligently directed one, under the control of the Vital Force of the whole organism. It cannot be haphazard or an unfortunate occurrence. The *Encyclopaedia Britannica* (14th ed., vol. 2) states:

The common idea of bacteria in the minds of most people is that of a hidden and sinister scourge lying in wait for mankind. This popular conception is born of the fact that attention was first focused upon bacteria through the discovery some 70 years ago, of the relationship of bacteria to disease in man, and that in its infancy the study of bacteriology was a branch of medical science. Relatively few people assign to bacteria the important position in the world of living things that they rightly occupy, for it is only a few of the bacteria known today that have developed in such a way that they can live in the human body, and for every one of this kind there are scores of others which are perfectly harmless and far from being regarded as the enemies of mankind, must be numbered among his best friends. It is, in fact, no exaggeration to say that upon the activities of bacteria the very existence of man depends; nay more, that without bacteria there could be no other living thing in the world; for every animal and plant owes its existence to the fertility of the soil and this, in turn, depends upon the activity of the micro-organisms which inhabit the soil in almost inconceivable numbers.

The writer of this article begins to show some understanding of the role of bacteria in the life processes. Bacteria are present universally and without them there would be nothing but sterility and death. Bacteria are normal and, even when particular bacteria are present as part of a particular disease process of the body, may be said to be normal for that process but *not* the primary cause of it. In the way that pain may be the *result* of a severe contraction of muscles, but not the cause of it, so then may bacteria be the *result* of a particular change in the body's chemistry, but not the cause of it. The bacteria are therefore a "normal" aspect of a total abnormality, of which bacterial activity is an identifiable part.

If an understanding of disease is built upon the view that

9

the life processes are largely chemical in nature, and not vital, then it will follow that the therapeutic approach to healing will also be chemical. Indeed, this belief is the cornerstone of conventional medicine which operates on the principle that, if you kill off the bug, then you get the patient well. Nothing could be further from the truth. The notion that it is possible to change a disease condition to a normal healthy one by assaulting the body with an assortment of chemicals designed to influence the perceived cause—bacteria or viruses—is almost medieval in concept.

Yet vast sums are spent to persuade us that it is so, that there is now a new drug which does not have the disadvantages of the last one, that it has been proven so much more effective in this or that condition; and so it goes on year after year. But perhaps the most important effect of all this is to persuade us that *the* cause of all these acute, infectious, illnesses often of unknown origin, is bacterial in origin and that this *must* involve antibacterial drug therapy. Anyone doubting such a proposition must be at best of lightweight intellect! If it is proven that bacteria are present in an illness, what other approach need there be?

It appears that hardly anyone has considered the possibility that germs—whether identified as bacteria or viruses— are only a part of the disturbance within the organism, a disturbance that arises from a dysfunction of the whole organism. The abnormal bacterial activity, which accompanies what we call "infections" or "infectious processes" but which is only one small indicator of abnormality, was made more prominent by advancing technology. We were mesmerized by the life-forms found to exist at the other end of the microscope; even more so, the electron microscope. We could see bacterial abnormality in the presence of particular disease syndromes and, therefore, the obvious equation between the two. Bacteria, it was concluded, must therefore be the cause of many of the infectious illnesses. There were some awkward questions to be answered nevertheless; such as, how is it that it is possible to find bacteria without there being any disease present?

The presence or absence of bacteria became the final determinant in arriving at a confirmed diagnosis. Without such information, the appellation of the name of an illness, such as tuberculosis, pleurisy, or typhoid, was merely guesswork. But, in all such cases, the presence of the specific bacterial organism was explicitly regarded as the offending or causative agent. That being so, it logically followed—so we were told—that if the offending bacteria could be destroyed, so then the whole disease process would be stopped. The tool to achieve this became the antibacterial drugs.

This is still the picture today. Drugs—sometimes bought off the shelf, sometimes prescribed—are designed to kill germs. The doctor writes the prescription to clear little Jimmy's runny nose—due to a virus; to take care of Mary's upset tummy—there is a bug going around; or to clear Richard's ongoing ear discharge—he keeps catching this infection. It is a doleful commentary on the level of understanding of even some of the most commonplace disorders like coughs and colds that so many of us are conditioned to believe that disorders such as these are somehow or other due to a bug on the loose. Our misunderstanding is compounded by the belief that the situation *must* call for the use of a drug appropriate to that particular disease organism.

We continue to look at a tiny fraction of the problem without appreciating that it may only be one aspect of a greater and integrated process being produced, choreographed, and directed by the body's unerring and omniscient self-correcting mechanisms. Even in the presence of disease processes, these self-correcting processes will continue to function to the best of that organism's ability. We must not forget that, in the presence of illness, the body's innate healing and reconstructive forces are all the while doing their utmost to resolve matters and to produce normality. This principle applies even in the presence of the gravest pathological deterioration such as with malignancy. The organism is striving to reverse abnormality even when apparently being overwhelmed. To introduce into this delicate situation a manufactured and destructive batch of chemicals is, for the most part, nothing but crass ignorance.

It is now probably quite impossible to make an objective assessment of the harmful effects—both short term and long term, and throughout populations—of this ongoing practice of aiming drugs at curing infections or viral-based diseases. One can only guess that the onslaught on the body's normal and natural processes over a period of years, and even generations, is likely to be harmful. Because of the underlying lack of philosophy of the champions of drug therapy and the resultant attempt to supplant the body's healing processes, it would seem possible, if not probable, that we risk changing the type and nature of one illness into that of another, a kind of mutational change in which one "disease" is substituted for another. For nature cannot be beaten and will always have the last laugh.

The Immune System

Frequent reference is now made in the general press and media, as well as the medical press, to the immune system. This has been largely, though not entirely, due to the alarming spread of AIDS—acquired immunodeficiency syndrome—a description of a particular group of symptoms which are serious and life threatening. The rather fulsome wording of the disease, when examined, means that it is attributed to a weakness, a shortfall of the body's normal ability to ward off threat or attack from microbial sources; that there is a weakness on the part of the body's normal immune system which is somehow or other "acquired."

Although reference to the immune system is made with increasing frequency, I am not sure that anyone has defined what the system actually is or consists of. It is not a readily identifiable system such as the circulatory system or the endocrine system or the genitourinary system. The immune system appears to be conveniently left without definition and therefore capable of interpretation as desired.

Immunity is defined in medical dictionaries as "security against any particular disease or poison, specifically, the power which an individual sometimes acquires to resist and/or overcome an infection to which most or many of its species are susceptible." The definition itself suggests an understanding of immunity which is tentative and inconstant. Any or all of the bodily systems which are involved in maintaining an infection-free organism are therefore part or parts of the immune system. It follows, then, that the presence of microorganisms would indicate infection and, therefore, a failure in some degree on the part of some constituents of the immune system.

One of the difficulties of the germ theory, however, is that microorganisms are often present without there being any evidence of illness. Thus in apparently healthy individuals, it is quite possible to find bacteria such as streptococcus, commonly attributed as being the cause of throat troubles, or staphylococcus, attributed as being the cause of some gastric disorders. The awkward question is, of course, if streptococcus is the cause of throat infections, why then does not everyone who has streptococcus present suffer from throat infections? If the immune system is intended to counteract these invasive organisms and has not done so, then presumably it has failed in some way. But if microorganisms can develop due to a weakened immune system, without there being any evidence of illness, what is the point of giving antibacterial drugs when symptoms do appear? After all, it is clear that the cause was with the weakened immune system and not the bacteria, otherwise the latter would *always* produce the symptoms of that illness. Shouldn't we therefore be trying to do something about helping the body's immune system to do its job, rather than firing off volley after volley of drugs at the bacteria?

But back to the question: What is the immune system? To the orthodox medical profession it is largely confined to matters of the blood and the integrity of its constituent components of red and white cells; associated with this will be the level of function of bone marrow tissue and of organs such as the spleen and liver. Closely linked with the integrity of the blood supply is the lymphatic system, which is really a part of the circulatory system and which is concerned with the important task of breaking down foreign bacteria.

Such a concept of the immune system is a very narrow one and concerns itself with the bacteriological abnormalities associated with particular disease syndromes. It is based upon the false assumption that the microscopically identifiable organisms are, *per se*, the cause of a variety of diseases. It excludes any consideration of the possibility that the microorganisms may be the *result* of the disease process rather than the cause of it. It also fails to recognize the possibility that the development of microorganisms can only take place in the presence of a weakened immune system and cannot—even with transmittable infections—take place in the presence of a healthy one. Indeed if this is so, then the immune system itself must be something more than just the blood, circulatory system, and associated structures.

Immunity from destructive and harmful forces, whether from within the body or without, can only be conferred within the context of total and integrated bodily function, and, of course, within the parameters required for survival, such as acceptable external temperature, adequate nutrition and fluid intake, absence of noxious materials such as chemicals and gases in the atmosphere, and so on. Some of these factors, it must be acknowledged, are of increasing and significant influence. But we are again here concerned, however, with the issue of function, with that balance required of our own bodily function in order that the myriad processes taking place within the body are doing so to their maximum potential. To delve into the minutiae of every bodily activity, every chemical procedure which takes place every second, every minute of every hour is likely to be of minimal value in furthering our knowledge of the health and disease processes, if it is divorced from the vitalistic view that the human organism is one integrated and interdependent series of activities all acting within the guidance of the body's innate intelligence, the Life Force. No cell is an island; no organ is an island; no system is an island. And the immune system has to be the totality of all the body's functions and systems. It is not a part; it is everything working in harmony. It performs a function which is the essence of the survival of the organism and, as such, must embrace the functional activities of the total life processes. Any disturbance to any function, any system is a disturbance to the immune system.

In such a light the folly of the antibacterial approach, by the use of drugs, will be clear. Not only is it based on a falsely conceived microbiological view of the body's reaction to threat, but it is likely to be harmful to the very processes required by the body to deal with such disturbance. The ravages to the body, over successive generations, as a result of a blind adherence to the antibacterial drug approach are quite impossible to estimate. This approach has continued unabated throughout this century and has grown worse, rather than better since the advent of the antibiotics. No one knows what subtle changes have been brought about in the form of, for example, chromosome changes, disturbances to essential enzymes, or an inability to adequately complete vital chemical changes in the system. To pinpoint and co-relate such matters causally would be infinitely more difficult than finding one's way out of the Amazon without a compass, for it highlights again the indisputable fact that all functions in the body are interdependent and incredibly complex. We are left therefore only to ponder and surmise the possible long-term consequences of what amounts to meddling with such sophisticated, yet delicate, processes.

The spread of AIDS disease is the latest in a long line of illnesses which are now impaled in the general consciousness as being attributable to a microorganism, in this case a virus which goes by the name HIV. Indeed, the illness perfectly illustrates my argument that the HIV virus is found to be present in numbers of people who do not suffer from AIDS. The virus is capable of transmission from one person to another, especially through sexual contact, but not everyone who has been in contact with an HIV virus "carrier" or AIDS sufferer appears to contract the virus.

And so the worldwide resources of the pharmaceutical industry are now harnessed toward the objective of either (a) killing off the virus, or (b) (potentially more profitable) producing a vaccine which will give "immunity" to those "at risk"; that is, the sexually active. What a lucrative prospect! Of course, this is a well-trodden path. As I have already suggested, the remedies being sought will, by their very nature, be likely to contribute to further weakening of the immune system which, in the case of AIDS, is even acknowledged by the name given it to be a disorder of the (narrow medically defined) immune system.

There is again not the slightest thought given to any other

possible reasons for the onset of the disease or of reasons why the immune system is weakened. The post-World War II upsurge in the incidence of venereal diseases was tackled with great gusto by the use of the new wonder drugs, the antibiotics, and continues apace. Has this practice in any way contributed to the artificial suppression of the venereal disease traits and changed the nature and character of them into another form, AIDS? And in what layer of the stratosphere did our little army of HIVs lurk these past millennia before deciding to strike? In any case, isn't it a silly notion that a healthy immune system can be knocked out of commission by a virus?

In AIDS, as in the whole theory of the bacteriological cause of disease, it will be necessary to rethink the premises upon which the current approaches of orthodoxy are based. We can be sure that the initiative will not come from the drug houses. We must look to saner people who are alerted to the destructive path along which we are traveling.

Insofar as I believe the body's defense mechanisms, its so-called immune system, to be the composite total of all functions, then the efficiency of that system must ultimately depend upon the level of function of the central controlling mechanism, the Unit of Function. What is meant by the Unit of Function is described in Chapter 7. It is the failure or partial failure at the level of this whole and central controlling mechanism which, above all else, *predisposes* the organism to systemic breakdown and allows invasive bacteriological forces to develop, either from within or without. It is the functional efficiency of this vital and protective system which will ensure survival and normality, not the overwhelming antilife forces embodied in the products of the pharmaceutical industry. The elephant has run amok in the china shop for too long.

Chapter 3

Symptoms

Symptoms are an indication that there has been a change from normal function to abnormal, either physically or mentally. They are therefore indicators, measurements by which we can assess that there has been a significant change for the worse in some area of bodily function. But symptoms are *not* the cause of the disorder or disease; they are the effect. So, the swollen and painful first toe joint is a symptom; the onset of a deeply depressive state is a symptom; the severe chest pain on walking upstairs is a symptom. As a rule it is when symptoms develop and persist that we seek medical advice and assistance, and it is assumed that before the symptoms arose everything was normal: We were healthy, or so we thought.

Symptoms are also generally regarded as being of some substance when they are reasonably specific and definable, such as those mentioned above. In such cases we *know* that something is wrong. The extent of the subjective departure from what we had hitherto taken to be normal was sufficiently marked as to leave no doubt that a change for the worse had taken place. This would be especially so if the change is sudden or occurs over a very short time span and/or if the change is accompanied by marked discomfort or pain.

On the other hand, symptoms may be of slow development. Our patient with the painful toe may have had little else to begin with other than an occasional and fleeting sense of a tingling sensation or slight pricking. This will have probably been dismissed as being nothing more than a mild nuisance caused by the last pair of shoes he bought. At that stage, the initial transient sensation will not have been considered to be a symptom in any real sense of the word. The need to seek medical help will not have arisen.

Yet the initial warning signals will at some stage cross the threshold, to be transformed from "nonsymptoms" to symptoms: It's time to do something. The early indications of abnormality, however slight, are nevertheless to be considered as symptoms and are still a sign that there has been some deviation from normal even though, in practice, it is quite understandable that medical help is not sought at that stage. For one thing, short-lived discomforts come and go, and do not always recur.

And then we have the abnormalities which are so trivial as to be dismissed altogether and are regarded as just something to be lived with. In this category we might find such things as a recurring hangnail on one finger; a skin wart that has been there ever since childhood; or, perhaps, a constantly blocked-up nostril. Such minor aberrations usually do not change over a period of many years and are not identified in the mind of the individual concerned as being an abnormality of their health in a substantive way.

In the strictest sense, therefore, anything which is recognizably a deviation from normal—and that includes what are termed a range of psychogenic symptoms—is an indication of abnormality and should be regarded as such by a physician, however dismissive a patient may be: "But I'm not concerned about the hangnail, Doc. I just want to get rid of this pain in my shoulder." So that taking the strict view of abnormality to include all the symptoms which are possible to manifest, few people go through a day, a week, a month without there being present *some* symptoms.

Symptoms, whether they are major or minor, have particular characteristics which are descriptive of the dysfunction or illness with which they are associated. These characteristics become the basis for appending to the symptom or group of symptoms, what then becomes the medical diagnosis for the illness; that is, the name of the disorder or disease. Mrs. A suffers from swelling and stiffness of the joints of the hands, fingers, and feet, with some degree of wasting of the muscles and is diagnosed as suffering from rheumatoid arthritis, a name which is descriptive of a particular group of symptoms. If, therefore, the symptoms fit the description of a particular disease category, the diagnosis is then determined accordingly.

If symptoms A = Disease A, then Diagnosis = Disease A

The investigation of the symptoms may involve simple or complex procedures, depending upon the nature of the symptoms, and much could be said about the need for and usefulness of many of them. This is due, in part at least, to the conditioning process which we have been subjected to, whereby we *expect* to have a name given to the illness from which we suffer. We also expect that the fullest investigation will be made commensurate with the nature and severity of the illness, including procedures which will exclude what might be deemed to be certain possibilities. The expectation is that once the diagnosis has been made—that is, the name has been given to the illness—the difficult part is over and the easier part, the resolution of the problem, is about to begin.

In a minority of cases, the nature of the dysfunction or illness will result in the symptoms clearing with or without medical treatment. This would apply to minor muscular pains and acute illnesses like common cold or influenza. But for the vast majority of chronic illnesses which result in persistent symptoms of one kind or another, there is a poor record of resolution from conventional medical treatment. This applies to a wide area of medical conditions such as skin problems, arthritic diseases, gastric disorders, general muscular-type pains, including neuritis disturbances such as sciatica, female disorders, cardiac and bronchial problems, all of which constitute a major proportion of everyday complaints in any medical facility.

The characteristics of any and each of these disorders are indicated by their symptoms, which in turn will determine the line of investigation to be followed—the diagnosis—which will result in the name of the disease. Many of these so-called diseases—perhaps more accurately described as collections of symptoms or symptom complexes—are then treated directly on the bases of the symptoms presented. For example, a skin condition will typically be treated externally by the use of creams or ointments which are applied direct to those areas of the body affected. The application of a cream in this way is to treat a symptom—an effect rather than a cause—and the type of cream will itself be determined by the diagnosis of the condition; that is, the name of the skin disease.

Symptoms A = Disease A = Cream A
Symptoms B = Disease B = Cream B, but not Cream A

This is referred to as symptomatic treatment: the treatment of symptoms, the treatment of effects and not causes. The basis of medical treatment is now almost entirely symptomatic as will a consideration of a few common everyday disorders indicate.

Frozen Shoulder Syndrome

This is a commonly found muscular disorder which results in pain, with restriction and limited movement of the shoulder joint. It is sometimes diagnosed as rheumatism, a very unspecific term in any case; and the treatment offered is usually some form of direct electrically based therapy to the shoulder area or, in more severe cases, steroid-based injections to the shoulder joint capsule. There is no attempt made to discover any possible cause, and so treatment is directed solely to the effect.

Hiatus Hernia

Again this is a terminology to describe a group of symptoms which arise from a disturbance in the area of the junction of the esophagus, the tubelike structure which carries the food from the mouth, where it enters the stomach. The main symptoms are discomfort and a burning sensation in the upper abdominal area, often aggravated by certain items of food. Inflammation is also usually present. The commonly prescribed treatments are reflux suppressants and antacid drugs aimed at alleviating the irritating effects of the natural stomach fluids by influencing their acid/alkaline balance, and suppressing the reflux effect of these fluids from traveling back up the esophagus. Such treatment is again symptomatic, aiming solely to influence the locally disturbed area. There is no pretense that anything in the realm of cure is being attempted. The objective is purely to alleviate, to hold the line.

Gallstones

A common condition is for fatty-based deposits to form within the gallbladder into relatively hard masses, which we call "stones." They consist mainly of the well-known fatty substance called "cholesterol." Gallstones are frequently present in the gallbladder without there being any evidence—symptoms—that they are there. Many a one has gone to his or her grave with a gallbladder full of gallstones and didn't even know it. The symptoms that lead to the investigation which results in the discovery of gallstones may include complaints of a sense of bloating in the abdominal area, usually getting worse as the day progresses; persistent indigestion; nausea; some degree of jaundice; or, perhaps an episode of severe pain in the midabdominal area. These symptoms by no means always arise from the presence of gallstones, but they raise the possibility and, if it transpires that stones are present, the suggested procedure is invariably to surgically remove the gallbladder. The possibility of conservative treatment hardly ever arises. The symptoms are the *effect* of gallbladder disease; and, in this case, it is argued that the *cause* is gallbladder disease. Therefore, the treatment will be to remove the cause in order to clear the effect: symptoms.

But it is necessary to go further back along the line and ask the question, why is it that the gallbladder is not functioning properly or is diseased? The fatty material contained within the gallbladder, which is a hollow organ, is bile, a naturally fatty-based substance essential for efficient digestion. It is abnormal for the bile to precipitate out of fluid solution to form into concreted masses of stones. The real question is, why should this happen? What *predisposing* factors were there to allow such a disturbance to happen? The practice of surgically removing gallbladders is still one of treating symptoms and is therefore symptomatic treatment.

Surgery may be necessary in situations where the nature of the disorder is life threatening and when a particular structure, such as a heart valve, has become irreversibly damaged. Even in these cases it must be appreciated that, in most cases, the deterioration will have been ongoing for some time and, in all probability, could have been resolved at an earlier date with the correct treatment, thereby obviating the ultimate necessity for surgery. But, for the most part, surgery has become the preferred treatment for a range of disorders, which are usually quite capable of resolution without the drastic trauma of surgery and in which symptoms are directly treated—if that is the word—to the exclusion of any basic understanding of cause.

Among this category would be procedures such as the following.

Varicose veins removed
Hemorrhoids excised
Partial removal of sections of the bowel for nonmalignant
    conditions such as colitis
Cardiac bypass procedures
Hysterectomies
Joint replacements
Nasal polyps
Removal or other surgical treatment of spinal discs

Conditions such as these (and many more) are primarily the result of *predisposing* disturbances of the central Unit of Function and require to be understood on that basis. The treatment of symptoms is to continue to leave the underlying causative factors untouched with the result that the body will continue to function only with difficulty. It will be merely to attempt to patch up each group of symptoms as they arise, to paper over the ongoing cracks in the wall whilst the foundations of the house continue to subside. As often as not, what we succeed in doing is to shift the symptom pattern from one "illness" to another over a period of years.

Chapter 4

Function

I have already mentioned the Unit of Function. An understanding of function is essential to the holistic view of the human organism: If we ignore function, we are more likely to concentrate on symptoms rather than causes.

What, therefore, is function? It is clear that where there is life, there is function; and when life ceases to exist, so, too, does function.

Function may be thought of as existing on two levels. Firstly, there is what may be termed *voluntary* function, which is to say that our conscious and voluntary acts result in a functional exercise in some part of the organism. For example, we decide to take the car out of the garage, so we consciously activate in a given order various sets of muscles which will result in us picking up the car key, walking to the garage, opening the garage door, starting the car, and so on. All of these movements were brought about by conscious decision and resulting in systematic, controlled, and, above all, *coordinated* movements which fulfilled our original intention. We do these things daily, and take it all very much for granted.

Secondly, there is what may be called *involuntary* function. Our hearts continue to expand and contract, supplying the body with essential blood and nutrition; but we don't need to be consciously involved in the process. We are not consciously required to take part in the liver's detoxifying processes; nor are we required to play an active part in filtration processes taking place in the tubules of the kidneys; nor do we need to be actively involved in the transportation of nutrients across the membranous walls of the millions of cells in the body.

We play no conscious part in effecting the involuntary processes; and yet they take place nonstop within each and every one of us from birth, even from conception, until death. These involuntary processes are as yet beyond the full knowledge or comprehension of science; they involve a myriad of processes affecting every cell, all tissues, all organs, and all systems of the body. The interplay of activities and the interdependence of functions is a miracle of timing, of assessment of needs and consequential provision of them. It is like imagining on a much vaster and complex scale the activity in an anthill, which we can be delighted with on our television screens, whereby the overall requirements of the organism of the anthill are somehow or other provided for *exactly* by all of the participants in the field of play.

Likewise, the participants in our own field of play are so hugely complex that it stretches our inadequate thought processes to begin to comprehend even a fraction of what is taking place. It is truly a part of the miracle of life, but how is it controlled? Or who or what does the controlling?

Such questions bring us to what, in many ways, are fundamental divergences of philosophy between the orthodox school of medicine, with its heavy emphasis on what it calls medical science, and the alternative therapies such as chiropractic, osteopathy (in its European form), homeopathy, acupuncture, and others. I think I am being fair and accurate when I say that orthodox medicine does not in any way see a *vital* factor in the functioning processes, but rather tends to see the human organism in terms of a complex chemical laboratory, the secrets of which will be largely unlocked by increasingly sophisticated biochemical investigations.

The alternative therapies, on the other hand, tend to

accept the broad principle that all life, including that of Man, is itself a manifestation of a greater principle, of a greater intelligence perhaps of a spiritual dimension. It is an understanding that accepts the nature of a process of such complexity and profundity that mere *Man* is never likely to understand in any total or chemical sense. The involuntary—and the voluntary for that matter—function is the very essence of the life processes, it is of such specificity, it is of such profound balance that, at the microcosmic level of cellular and biochemical activity we are left gasping at its enormity.

In contradistinction to the biochemical one, such an understanding is looked upon as a *vitalistic* one, based upon the premise that all function and all activity is entirely governed and controlled by the Vital Force which, itself, may be described as a constructive, self-regulating, self-correcting principle permeating all living matter. It is intangible; it cannot be measured and yet its "dynamic" is the essence of all living activity. Such a subtle concept continues to be ignored by modern science, but yet remains at the core of the various alternative healing schools. The chiropractors refer to it as the "Innate"; Samuel Hahnemann, the founder of the homeopathic school, called it the "Dynamis"; Claude Bernard referred to it as the "Life Force," and Henri–Louis Bergson as the *"Elan Vital."*

I leave the last word on the issue of Vitalism to Professor T. J. Lyle, A.M., M.D., whose quaint writings are as true today as they were when he wrote in 1896: "To aid the vital force in these restorative efforts is the work of true medicine from the hands of a true physician." And, again: "The physical basis of life is vital and not chemical. The conservation of the vital force is the pivotal point in therapeutics." Lyle states, "By virtue of this vital force and living matter the body is able to maintain its *functional integrity* [my emphasis] against ordinary adverse influences" (1896).

Chapter 5

Functional Interdependence

It is clear that functional integrity means functional coordination, if it means anything. By that I mean that no activity taking place within the organism is independent or stands alone or does not influence or is not influenced by other activities. It is a balance.

Let us make an assumption. Let us assume that the human organism was designed by an omniscient Engineer in such a way that it would purr through life like a Rolls Royce car without a squeak and without a sign of failure. Such an assumption may seem difficult to allow, given the widespread evidence of breakdown all around; but it would seem reasonable, nevertheless, to suppose that, somehow, the potential for such an optimum state of affairs exists among the apparent complexities of anatomy and physiology.

If we had such a finely tuned individual, firing 100 percent on all cylinders, at any given moment in time there are, as we have already considered, billions of physiological activities, voluntary and involuntary, taking place simultaneously and each having an influence one upon the other. What, then, might be the interdependence between such a person's stomach and, say, the first toe?

Well, the stomach receives blood and, therefore, nutrients to maintain the health of its own cells.

The nerve supply to the stomach plays a part in the movement of food from the time it is swallowed until the time it leaves to pass into the intestine. This utilizes the muscles of the lining of the stomach.

The glands of the stomach in turn act to provide the mechanism whereby the food is to be broken down and the nutrients assimilated to be returned to the blood supply for transportation around the body.

Now, the first toe, like all tissue, requires nutrition which, as we have seen, involves, among other things, adequate nutrition brought through by the blood supply. It also, for optimum health, requires adequate drainage to clear waste products.

In such a simple model we can readily see that any factor which would disturb stomach function in such a way as to affect its ability to assimilate and transport nutrients to the blood supply would ultimately have *some* detrimental effect on the big toe, because the level of nutrition available to it would be indirectly disturbed at the stomach level.

Thus, it is established that disturbed *function* at the stomach level will have a deleterious effect on the first toe. The toe, however, is not going to indicate that there is any disturbance. It is not necessarily going to produce any symptoms such as pain, wasting of muscles, inflammation (watch out for the virus here!) or gangrene. No, indeed; and it is very likely that the departure from a level of optimum nutrition, brought about in turn by a diminution in stomach function, will continue without there appearing in the toe any group of symptoms to indicate all is not as it should be.

The foregoing example of interdependence is intended to indicate the relationship that exists between function at the level of any major system or organ, on the one hand, and function at an area of the body apparently unconnected with, and often geographically remote from, the other. To mix a metaphor, "No cell is an island." But it also highlights the confusing question of the appearance of symptoms.

This example of a connection between the stomach and toe can be related ad infinitum to include function between practically any one part of the body and any other. The possible permutations on this theme are endless but, if nothing else, consideration of this question of interrelationship and interdependence becomes focused and sharpened in our consciousness, lest we lose sight of both the existence and importance of such factors. For we otherwise risk being whisked along in a river of medical jargon which has long since lost sight of such concepts in its search to "see with what avidity medical men have allowed themselves to run after therapeutical sensations." We shall return in due course to the question of symptoms as part of our attempt to reach an understanding about disease causation.

Chapter 6

Nerve Function

The role of the nervous system is probably not fully appreciated in relation to the part it plays in maintaining the body's integrity; that is, health. There is a widespread view, for example, that certain characteristics exhibited by some people have, in some way, to do with their "nerves." The excitable are believed to be so because that's the way they are and that is always the way they have been; such characteristics have therefore something to do with their "mind." The same view would be taken of other categories, such as the depressive, weepy person who really only needs to pull himself together because it's all in the "mind." At the other end of the spectrum, there is the apparently brave or daring type who is deemed to "not have a nerve in his body."

All of these views reflect an understanding of a relationship between nerves and the mind; and that the latter is, for the most part, a reflection or aspect of personality—which is to say that it is therefore unalterable; that it is part of the person, of the personality; that it is etched in stone. If and when such characteristics ever assume magnified proportions to the point where they might be considered intolerable, either by the person concerned or by family or friends, then that person is deemed to have an illness which has something to do with the nerves. In reality it is meant that it has something to do with the mind, an area of our being which is in any case difficult to define.

Another group of illnesses associated with nerve disorders are those which display a marked physical group of symptoms and which manifestly involve nervous tissue. In this group would be included chronic and degenerative illnesses such as multiple sclerosis and parkinsonism. There are clear and well-defined symptoms, certainly as such illnesses progress, associated with the body's nerve function; and we consider these to be diseases of the nervous system; that is, of nerve tissue.

Probably the other major groups of illnesses are those of an acute nature, where there is often evidence of inflammation present (viruses?). Here we would include illnesses such as sciatica, shingles, and tic douloureux; and once again the evidence is clear of disturbance of a physical nature to nerve tissue.

In all of these types of illnesses, there is considered to be overt and clear evidence of dysfunction of some area of the nervous system, whether it be of, say, psychological origin, as from the mind, or whether it be physical. As a general rule it is considered that, in the absence of any of these types of illnesses, that major controller of so much of all bodily functions, the nervous system, which exercises such vast control over practically every function in our bodies, is otherwise normal and functioning satisfactorily.

But is it? Nerve dysfunction or disturbance is presumed to be absent if there are no clear signs or symptoms of the nervous system itself, such as in the foregoing types of conditions. In other words if there are no symptoms, we accept that normality prevails, which means that nerve control and function are at full or optimum level. This is very much a case then of black or white, either/or: *Either* there is clear disease often with accompanying changes of nerve tissue, *or* all is entirely normal. There are no shades of gray in between. Can things be so black or white?

The specific purpose of nerves is simply to transmit and receive signals. Even the microchip has a long way to go before it could ever hope to match the efficiency and complexity of Man's computer. All tissue is designed to allow it to comply with the specific function for which it is designed, and so nerve tissue has its specialty in the particular purpose of sending and receiving messages. This, then, is the *function* of nerve tissue. There are few other functions of the body, from those associated with the health and workings of the major organs and systems down to microscopic biochemical interactions, with which the nervous system is not vitally involved; and so, in practice, nerve function is frequently an essential prerequisite to other bodily functions.

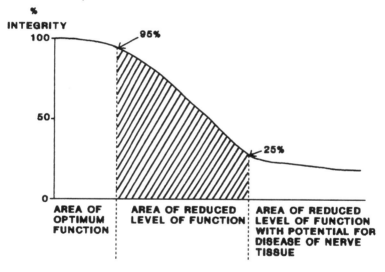

Fig. 1. Graph of Nerve Function

In Figure 1 I have shown a theoretical and arbitrary diagram designed purely to illustrate the point that there is frequently, at any given time in any given person, a level of efficiency of nerve function which may be anywhere between the optimum possible, at one end of the scale, to a very much reduced level at the other. Anything which represents a level of efficiency of less than 100 percent is strictly abnormal; but from a purely practical point of view, it is being allowed that anything down to, say, 95 percent is acceptable and may be regarded as normal.

At the other end of the scale, it is suggested that anything below, say, 25 percent of normal function has reached the stage of being potentially at a point where frank and recognizable disease of the nervous system is possible. This would include the chronic group of illnesses previously referred to, such as parkinsonism and severe neuralgias.

In between these two groups, in the shaded part, is a large area where we have little evidence of nerve dysfunction *per se*, and yet it is in this area that much disturbance lies. The problem here is that we are conditioned to believe that normality exists except when symptoms are present. We do not think that abnormality can exist without symptoms being present; not surprising when for so long it has been implicit in our approach to medicine that you have to have particular and newly acquired symptoms before you go to see the doctor; or you have few or moderate or no symptoms and therefore you are well and don't need to see the doctor. It is only in relatively recent years that the notion of what we call preventive medicine has taken hold and that it might be of value to have health checkup, even though there are no symptoms present.

This gray area of reduced or inefficient function, which is widespread, is of the utmost importance, however. Nerve function is an essential part of just about every process being carried on in our bodies throughout every second, minute, hour, and day of our lives. It is required to ensure proper function both at the voluntary and involuntary level. For example, the hollow structures such as arteries and intestines are all lined with muscular tissue, which of course expands and contracts constantly (Fig. 2a). That is the nature of

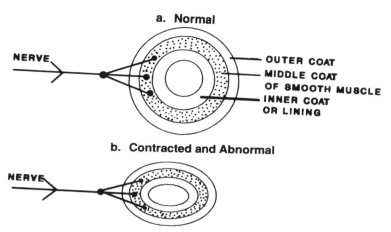

Fig. 2. Cross Section of Typical Artery

muscular tissue; but the expansion and contraction processes are controlled entirely by the nervous system. Muscular tissue is as nothing unless the nervous system is telling it what to do. In the case of an artery, it is quite possible for there to be disturbances to its nerve supply which will result in a contraction or tightening of the middle coat of smooth muscle of a permanent nature; in such circumstances the smooth muscle is unable to fully relax. The result of permanent contraction of some degree (Fig. 2b) is that the profile of the artery, which is essentially a hollow tube, is compressed. And if the tube is compressed, it will follow that fluids flowing through it—in this case, blood—will be decreased in volume. Since blood is the major source of nutrients for cells, it will follow that, in such a scenario, the nutrition to those cells being supplied by this particular artery will be reduced accordingly. An end effect like this would, let us not forget, have its origin in a failure of function of the nervous system in the first instance.

Another area of bodily function which we might usefully consider is the effect of the nervous system in the performance level of a major organ. The liver, for example, is a very complex organ, playing a very important role in the body's metabolism. Once again the nervous system is a crucial actor in the overall performance level of such an organ and will have at the very least a significant effect on all those vital functions required to sustain overall health of the body. It can be seen from Figure 3 that nerve control of the liver plays an essential part in determining the ability of the organ in turn to carry out some of its important tasks. If, however, there is some element of disturbance to the transmission mechanism of the nerve impulses supplying the liver, it can be seen that there is a likelihood, if not certainty, of that disturbance being reflected in some or all of those functions carried out by the organ.

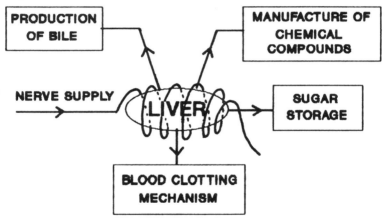

Fig. 3. Liver Function

In these two examples, important and vital processes required to sustain general health—the transportation of adequate blood and, therefore, nutrients to cells in one case; and in the other, the manufacture of complex chemical substances, the facility of storing of sugars, the production of bile for digestive purposes, and the provision of elements required to allow clotting of the blood—all these and much more—are dependent above all else on the integrity and efficiency of the nervous system.

Any disturbance to nerve *function* will have its resultant disturbance in equal measure to the *function* of any organs or other bodily systems with which that section of the nervous system is associated. Which brings us back again to that gray area of dysfunction of the nervous system in which there is neither full and efficient function nor recognizable and evident dysfunction or even disease. And, if there is such an area of dysfunction at the level of the nervous system, then it seems reasonable to suppose that we are likely to have a similar gray area of dysfunction at the tissue and organ level throughout the body.

Chapter 7
The Unit of Function

Two of the major healing philosophies in the world of natural healing originated in the United States. These were the disciplines of chiropractic and osteopathy. Both produced much reaction and opposition from the establishment of the day—and still do. Both were concerned with the relationship between the structure of the body, especially of the spine, and bodily function. Spinal mechanics was perceived as being within the field of both professions; and it was also understood, in spite of the philosophical writings of the early developers, that both therapies were increasingly concerned with neuromusculoskeletal (NMS)-type conditions to the exclusion more and more of "medical"-type illnesses such as angina, colitis, or duodenal ulcer. And so, today, a patient would commonly decide to consult a chiropractor or osteopath to seek help with an NMS-type condition; but only relatively rarely would such a professional be sought to help with a medical-type problem.

All of this arose because the fundamental cornerstone of thinking of both professions lay in the need for anatomical balance of the bones of the spine, misalignment of which was an important causative factor in the production of a wide range of painful conditions involving nerves—for example, sciatica—and the musculature, often otherwise vaguely diagnosed with nomenclature such as lumbago, slipped-disk syndrome, or just plain rheumatism.

In Figure 4, we see that the adult spine consists of twenty-six bones in all. These bones are each referred to as a

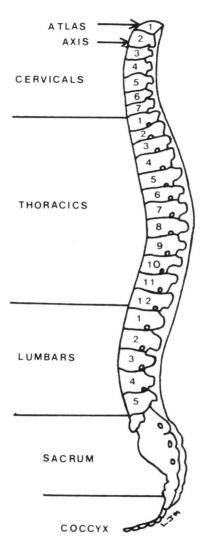

Fig. 4. The Spine

vertebra. The first, or upper, seven vertebrae, which basically constitute the neck, are called the cervical spine (Cl-C7). The next twelve are referred to as the thoracic spine (T1-T12), and below this are the five vertebrae (L1-L5) which constitute the lumbar spine. Below L5 is the sacrum which comprises five separate vertebrae until about the age of twenty-five by which time they are fused to form one wedge-shaped bone. And, finally, there is the coccyx which begins life as four or five separate vertebrae and which become fused in adulthood.

Associated with each vertebra are complex ramifications of nerves which are, in turn, distributed to various areas of the body and take part in just about every conceivable activity of physiology, both *voluntary* and *involuntary*. This may be in the activation of voluntary muscles in order to, say, walk or pick up a pencil or get up out of a chair. It may be concerned with the control of blood along the arteries in order to bring nutrition to, say, the tissue of a major organ such as the kidney; or it may be concerned with the complex work done by a major system such as the gastrointestinal.

It will be readily seen that there is a very decided relationship between the segments, or vertebrae, of the spinal column and nerve distribution, and that irregularities or disturbances at any level of the spinal column are therefore likely to lead to disturbed neurology. Since neurology, as we have seen, is crucially involved in various bodily functions, it seems reasonable to suppose that spinal irregularities (these were known as subluxations by the chiropractors and as lesions by the osteopaths) would lead directly to some element of functional impairment of the body's mechanisms. And so it was determined that any anatomical departure of any vertebra from what would be regarded as normal would have a deleterious effect on *function*. Any such analysis was based on the understanding that the spinal lesion was of the nature of a "mechanical" displacement, which is to say that the vertebrae are to a large extent considered to be independent of each other and that, although a lesioned or displaced or misaligned vertebra will to some extent affect other vertebrae, especially those most proximate to it, there is usually a vertebra that is central or primary to the problem. Such is still the view today of some practitioners.

In 1899 William Garner Sutherland, a student at the American School of Osteopathy in Kirksville, Missouri, had his attention directed to a disarticulated skull owned by Dr. A. T. Still, the founder of osteopathy. He became intrigued by the nature of the beveled articulations, or joints, between the bones of the skull, and so began thirty years of study, investigation, and research.

Contrary to popular belief, the human skull, or cranium, is not composed of one or two bones but consists of a total of twenty-three bones, if we exclude the small ossicles of the inner ears (Fig. 5). Sutherland believed that contained within the design of some of the beveled surfaces, which are really joints between bones, there existed the possibility of movement between the bones, thus allowing for the presence of a respiratory-type mechanism.

Such a concept ran counter to the accepted and established view that, in the adult, there is no movement of any of the cranial bones and that the articulations between the bones—called "sutures"—were indeed ossified.

Sutherland has been proven correct, but his discovery has been slow to gain acceptance and the full significance of it has scarcely been fully realized. The result has been that, although the cranium is now widely recognized within the professions as being of *some* overall significance in health care provision, there is not a general consensus as to its degree of importance in our understanding and treatment of either the NMS-type conditions or the wider general medical conditions.

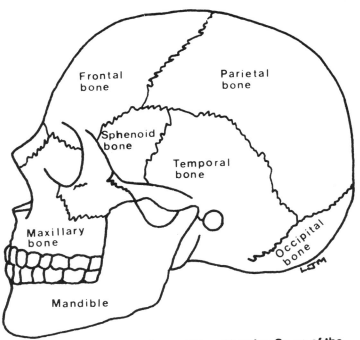

**Fig. 5. The Cranium: A Lateral View Showing Some of the
Larger Bones**

The cranium sits on top of the spine—or, the spine may
be said to hang from the cranium. The cranium is no more a
self-contained unit separate from the spine than the spine is
one, separate from the cranium. Indeed, the two are joined
anatomically in the area of the first cervical vertebra and the
occipital bone of the cranium. In any real sense the occipital
bone may be regarded as another vertebra, albeit of a different design, articulating with the first cervical vertebra just
as the second cervical vertebra does with the first, as the third
does with the second, and so on.

That there is a rhythmic, respiratory type of movement
of the bones of the cranium is now well established and the
existence of such an *involuntary* movement forms the basis of

the work currently being carried out in this area by practitioners from both disciplines; such skills are referred to as cranial osteopathy, or craniopathy. In practice, it is found that this respiratory movement, involving all the bones of the cranium, takes place at a rate of about ten to fourteen times per minute and is effectively one of motion between an alternating expansion and contraction phase.

The drive mechanism, or transmission shaft, of this respiratory movement occurs at the junction of two of the twenty-three cranial bones, these being the occipital and the sphenoid.

In Figure 6 these two bones are shown separately from the other bones of the cranium. During the respiratory movement, they move about a joint which may be thought of as a fulcrum. In Figure 6 the fulcrum is indicated by the arrow. The sphenoid is the bone to the left and the occipital the bone to the right. The amount of movement is, of course, very slight. The direction of the movement during the relaxation phase is indicated by the direction of the arrow in 6a. Note the relative position between the two bones at the fulcrum. The direction of movement during the contraction phase is shown in 6b and the relative position between the two bones should again be noted. The relative position of the occipital to the sphenoid changes at the fulcrum during these phases and, since there are articulations between every bone in the cranium and every adjacent bone at the sutures, or joints, it follows that there is movement of *all* cranial bones during this respiratory or involuntary rhythmic motion.

The cranium, which may be likened to a closed spherical ball made up of a number of joined units, therefore is a unit of motion which consists of processes of alternating expansion and contraction. It might be likened to a damp sponge which, when contracted or squeezed will slowly expand until squeezed again, with the process in the case of the cranium

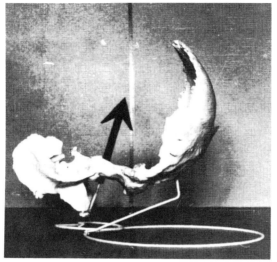

a. Relaxation Phase

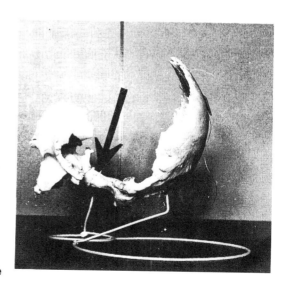

b. Contraction Phase

Fig. 6. Occiput/Sphenoid

continuing throughout life. This expansion and contraction process is a crucial factor in the provision and maintenance of the life processes. Such movement, or motility, has a number of effects within the cranium itself. For instance, it influences the movement of blood and oxygen into the head, the drainage of blood and waste products from the head, the production and movement of cerebrospinal fluid, and much else besides.

The origin of some 80 percent of the nervous system of the body, both the voluntary and involuntary systems, arises in the brain, which is, of course, within the cranial cavity. In relation to general bodily function at all levels, the essential control of the myriad functions which are required to sustain the life processes are effected by means of the nervous system. This, as we have seen, applies to both the *voluntary* and *involuntary* functions.

It is generally agreed among craniopaths that the origin of motion of the cranial bones lies in the brain itself. The brain, which constitutes so much of the nervous system, is like our sponge, continually contracting and expanding within self-limiting phases, the mechanism of which is not fully understood. It is, however, the constant changes of pressure within the cranial cavity brought about by the expansion and contraction of the brain which give rise to an alternating increase and decrease of pressure upon the cranial bones and which cause these in turn to move rhythmically and in harmony with the brain.

Thus, the brain is the engine of movement within the cranium and the origin of the *involuntary* movement of the cranial bones. What, then, is the significance of all this?

The brain is enclosed inside three layers of tissue called membranes. One of these membranes called the dura is attached to the internal walls of the cranium and extends out of the cranium in such a way as to cover and protect the spinal cord with its masses of nerve fibers. The dura finally attaches to and terminates at the sacrum which, apart from the first and second cervical vertebrae, is the only other vertebra to which the dura is connected.

This means that there is a physical connection between the cranium and the base of the spine. It also means that this connecting link between the cranium and the base of the spine (Fig. 7), which consists of a very strong fibrous material, will result in disturbances at one end of the dural terminations, be it at the sacrum or at the cranium, being transmitted to the other end. Stresses, strains, or disturbances of any kind at the sacral end of the dural tube will therefore have resultant stresses reflected at the cranial end of the tube. *And vice versa.*

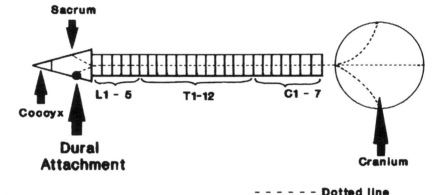

Fig. 7. The Dura

Looking again at the mechanism involved, we can see that we have the brain—the sponge—with its ongoing respiratory motion of contraction and expansion, producing the same motion on all the bones of the head, articulating as they do about the sutures. The movement will also be reproduced exactly at the base of the spine via the dura. We can perhaps visualize this as a wavelike movement, an ebbing and flowing, something akin to the movement of a snake through the grass. The movement will also include motion of all of the intermediate vertebrae in the spine, from top to bottom.

And so we have what might be called the Unit of Function; that is to say, the central controlling unit which makes us tick and upon which the essential bodily functions depend. This Unit of Function will basically comprise

1. the brain
2. the spinal cord
3. the cranium
4. the dura
5. all of the vertebra

Within this unit and under its control, the major physiological processes of the body take place. It follows that any disturbances to any part of this unit will have resultant disturbances to normal body function and, therefore, to health.

Chapter 8
Dysfunction

If we are alive, and we hope we are, then we are functioning. The level, or degree, of function will depend upon a number of factors, the most important and significant of which are (a) age and (b) the efficiency, or balance, of what I have called the Unit of Function.

In the case of the age factor, there will be a differing level of function taking place with all of our physiological processes directly related to age. This would be normal, of course, and therefore is excluded from our present considerations. While age itself is unalterable (other than by cheating on your birth certificate!), the process which we call "aging" is itself subject also to considerable influence by the second of these considerations.

The act of function is one of alternating expansion and contraction, a process which takes place throughout the whole of the constituent parts of our functional unit, and at the same level of function throughout. By that I mean that if the process of expansion and contraction is taking place at the source, or origin, of the mechanism—that is, the brain— then so will that same level of function be taking place throughout the unit. If this were expressed as a percentage, then if the level of function—expansion and contraction— taking place at the brain were 80 percent of what it ought to be, then that same reduced level of function at 80 percent of normal would apply to the unit in total. If the engine of the car is performing at only 80 percent of capacity, then the drive shaft is only doing the same.

So let us drop a monkey wrench into the works of this potentially flawless mechanical system. Let us suppose that the drive mechanism is somehow or other disturbed in such a way as to affect *function*. What then?

If we look at the constituent parts of our functional unit—the brain, the spinal column, the vertebrae, the dura, and the cranium—the only ones of these capable of being warped or displaced would appear to be either the cranium with its own semienclosed bony structure or the vertebrae. And we might also include the possibility of the large pelvic bone called the "innominate," since the sacrum articulates with it and might therefore be influenced by it. The brain and spinal cord are masses of nerve fiber, are not therefore by themselves likely to be strong enough to disturb the rhythmic expansion and contraction movement, whereas resistance at the bony level would.

It would certainly be reasonable to assume that any significant displacement (lesion) of any one or more of any of the vertebrae would introduce a stress factor, an embarrassment, into the efficient working of the unit. So, too, would any displacement of the innominate, with its direct articulation with the sacrum. In spite of all this, I do not believe that this is where the main source of dysfunction arises.

In any well-engineered and honed piston and cylinder arrangement, we might find a system of movement as in Figure 8. In 8a the piston is moved fully along the hollow cylinder to the left; and in the reverse movement in 8b, it is moved along the cylinder fully to the right. In this way the cylinder allows the piston to move back and forth to its maximum degree, and therefore the efficiency of the other functions for which this full and unobstructed movement of the piston is crucial is maximized.

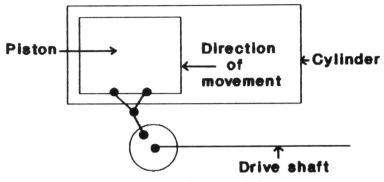

a. Piston Moved to Left

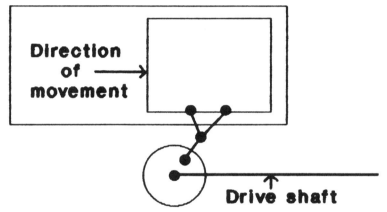

b. Piston Moved to Right

Fig. 8. Piston and Cylinder

Suppose, however, that the hollow cylinder developed a flaw, a warp; then the piston would be unable to move freely and the functional efficiency of the total movement would therefore be impaired as in Figure 9. The totality of the range of movement of the piston within the cylinder would be impaired, as would all those other functions which depended upon it.

We can now translate this analogy to our human functional unit, in which it is predicated that the efficiency of the rhythmic alternating motion will be adversely affected by a flaw, a warp in the bony structures of the unit. And, it is undoubtedly true, that any primary flaw in the bony components—the pillars of the edifice—will influence the range of motion which can take place as part of the alternating motion.

If, however, we look more closely, we can discern that the one area above all else which can and will have the most profound and significant effect on function is in the engine casing itself—the cranium.

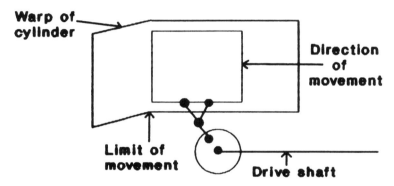

Fig. 9. Piston and Warped Cylinder

Chapter 9
Birth

We have seen that, of all the twenty-three bones which constitute the cranium, the two which are central to the whole driving momentum are the occipital and the sphenoid, two bones which are joined uniquely in such a way as to form a fulcrum.

The occipital and sphenoid (see Fig. 6) continue to alter their position in relation to one another in such a way that the angle at the fulcrum decreases during the expansion (relaxation) phase of motion (Fig. 10a) and increases during the contraction phase (Fig. 10b).

During this alternating movement of expansion and contraction, we must not lose sight of the fact that, while the occiput and sphenoid are the hub bones involved, the remaining bones of the cranium also move in their individual ways during each of the phases of expansion and contraction as part of a *total* movement. Nor must we lose sight of the movement of the dura, exactly replicating the movement of the cranial bones; and of the sacrum, replicating the movement of the dura; and, not least, of the vertebrae, replicating the effect on them of the occiput, the dura, and the sacrum. We have, in every conceivable way, a living, vibrant, constantly moving unit in which the harmony of the whole is dependent upon the parts.

If we refer back again to the cranium and consider the interdependence between the bones which is built into the design of this section of the unit, we can clearly see that any flaw, any misalignment of any one or more of the bones will

SPHENOID   **FULCRUM**   **OCCIPITAL**

Unbroken line ▪ neutral or mid position of sphenoid/ occipital

Broken line ▪ reduced angle at fulcrum during relaxation phase of movement

a. During Relaxation Phase

SPHENOID   **FULCRUM**   **OCCIPITAL**

Unbroken line ▪ neutral or mid position of sphenoid/ occipital

Broken line ▪ increased angle at fulcrum during contraction phase of movement

b. During Contraction Phase

Fig. 10. Movement of Sphenoid/Occipital

introduce a stress into the cranium in total. Which is to say that, if, as seems reasonable, the totality of motion of all of the cranial bones can only take place *at an optimum level* in the presence of a free, balanced, and properly positioned relationship of all bones, one with each other, then any alteration in that optimally positioned relationship will have an adverse effect on motion. Such disturbed motion at the cranium will, once again, have a similar effect on motion throughout those other constituent parts of the unit.

It is here that it becomes necessary to take a long, hard, and searching look at your ordinary everyday cranium; and this we will do presently. First, though, let us have a look at a cranium which does not confuse us with the trappings of life, such as with skin, hair, eyes, and so on. Let us for a moment look at a skull whose contours we can see clearly and which cannot lie. Let me introduce Henry (Fig. 11). If we look from behind (11a), we see the signs of an overall distortion of the bones, particularly evident in comparison of the two beveled surfaces A and B. B on the right is much lower than A. Other irregularities can be seen such as the more sloping surface of the left side at C as against the right side at D.

Looking at Figure 11b, where we view Henry from above and behind, we can see the marked evidence of the rotation of the midline point A to the left. This view also shows the bulge at B on the right side compared to the indentation on the same area on the left side at C. This gives a clear indication of the degree to which Henry is twisted, or rotated, in a clockwise direction. If we were to examine Henry in further detail, we would see clear evidence of other areas of gross misalignment which would be part of an overall pattern of distortion of the skull.

It is important to appreciate that Henry was not selected because he, exceptionally, exhibited the flaws indicated. The point here is that all skulls have some degree of distortion;

54

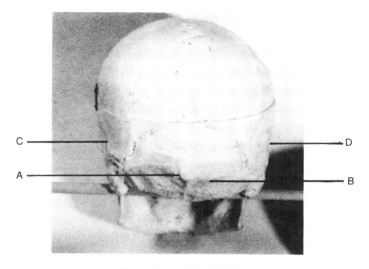

a. Bone Distortion Evident

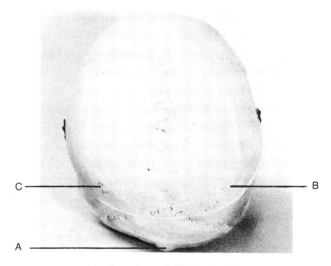

b. Rotation of Midpoint Line

Fig. 11. Henry

some worse, some better than Henry. And this brings us to the quite incredible realization that each one of us, at the cranial level, is in some degree of anatomical warp. This means, of course, that the mechanisms of movement, both within the cranium and of the bones themselves, are in some degree impaired. The piston and cylinder arrangement, involving the movement of the sphenoid and occiput, is no longer able to perform to the maximum, or optimum, level of efficiency, with all the consequences that entails for the functional unit in its entirety. And so how, you will ask, does such a state of affairs come about? How is it that practically all of us have some element of flaw, or distortion, of the cranial structure when the design is inherently flawless?

The answer to this question is one that still exercises those of us researching in this field, but would appear to be related in some way to the effects of birth. There are many factors surrounding not only the birthing process itself, but also the influences and forces on the uterus during the period of pregnancy. Much has been written in the technical journals about these matters by a relatively small number of practitioners who are interested in, and who recognize the importance of, the cranium in respect of the total health requirement.

But suffice to say that my own view is that there are particular and specific objectives to be met in order that the cranium ultimately assumes the ability to function at its maximum, or optimum, level. These objectives are not being achieved fully at or before birth for reasons which we do not yet fully understand; they appear to be in some part connected with the molding and decompression effects resulting from the infant's passage through the birth canal. But there are also, at least in some cases, influences on the unborn infant from intraabdominal pressures from the mother. Even, surprisingly, in the case of infants born following cesarean section of the mother, there are influences denied such children because of the failure to arrive in this world in nature's intended way.

The reasons for this rather extraordinary state of affairs are at present speculative and are the subject of what can only be described as inadequate and poorly funded research, largely because the importance of the issues involved is not recognized other than by the meagerest of numbers of practitioners. It is clear, however, that trauma from the birthing process does occur, even if it is unclear exactly how and why this is so. The weaknesses or distortions which we commonly find in the cranium have a significance which a craniopath finds difficult to overstate.

Recalling that the nervous system has a predominant influence on the health of individual organs and that the Unit of Function is the critical determinant of nerve function, we can conclude that distortions in the most important element of the Unit of Function—the cranium—have a pervasive and major effect on the health of the whole human organism. Let us now look at this in detail.

Chapter 10
Nerve Mechanisms

As part of the normal alternating, rhythmic movement of the nervous system—both that part of the system contained within the cranium and constituting the brain, and that part originating at the various segments of the spine—there is also movement or motion of other structures, including the bones of the cranium.

The powerhouse of all this motion appears to be within the brain itself, although the precise mechanism is not yet clear. It would also appear that the objective of the exercise is that this motion, which consists of alternating contraction and expansion of the brain, should be as free as possible. In other words the motion should be able to reach a maximum degree of movement as part of the expansion cycle and a maximum degree of movement as part of the contraction cycle. Such maximum motion will take place *providing there are no impediments or obstructions to influence it.*

But, unfortunately, there are. The major impediment to movement will be the bony casing surrounding the brain; and this bony casing (the cranial bones)—which moves synchronously with the internal engine, the brain—will be itself incapable of movement to its maximum degree because of the disturbance arising from birth or prebirth. This is something akin to a logjam of movement. The cranial bones are, in total, in some degree of asymmetry or warp, giving rise, in particular, to a restriction in the range of motion capable of being achieved by the sphenoid and occipital bones about their fulcrum. Such restriction in movement of these two bones to their opposite poles of motion will finally offer resistance to the range of motion—expansion and contraction—which the brain itself can achieve.

So what does all this mean from the point of view of its effects on general health? My own view is that there are a number of consequences to this which will result in negative effects to areas of our physiology such as the endocrine (hormonal glands) system and production of the cerebrospinal fluid within the brain. But probably the greatest area of influence is to the nervous system itself, bearing in mind all those many other activities of the body which are directly controlled in some degree by the nervous system.

For example, let us think back to muscular tissue which essentially has the task of contracting and relaxing, both at the voluntary and at the involuntary level. In the case of the voluntary muscular system, we activate those muscles required to allow us to embark on a particular task—say, get up out of the chair. Theoretically, when we are sitting in the chair and are in a totally nonactive, or relaxed, state, all voluntary muscles should be relaxed. In practice, however, it is found that voluntary muscle groups are almost always in some degree of contraction; that is, not completely relaxed. And this at times when, in theory at least, they should be. Why should this be so?

As we know, contraction and relaxation of such muscle groups is very largely determined by the nervous system; and it is to this system that we must look for answers to this phenomenon. A common finding in voluntary muscle disorders is that this inability of the muscle groups to become totally relaxed is always present, which means that there is a permanent level of built-in tightness or tension in the muscles which must be regarded as abnormal. At this point there is often very little indication of abnormality other than perhaps some element of minor restriction of movement or of stiffness, which is not *considered* by the sufferer to be abnormal. But abnormal it is, and such a situation represents a level of preexisting tension of tissue which will provide the foundation for the severe painful condition which arises commonly. This is often in the form of muscular spasm, sometimes with accompanying inflammation, and usually triggered off by some additional stress or contracting feature.

It has to be noted, however, that the preexisting contraction of the muscles resulted from some element of abnormality of nerve impulses. Remember, muscular tissue is nothing but inert flaccid flab capable of no activity until the nervous system provides its input. It cannot expand or contract without those vital messages from the nervous system. And so, if the muscular system is in some degree of overcontraction in the first instance—and this can only be caused by the nervous system—we have to ask ourselves, what has gone wrong at the nerve end of the muscular system?

We have to look for some departure from normal of nerve *function*. We are back again into the gray area of a drop-off of nerve function but without there necessarily being frank nerve disease itself. And, if there is a reduction in nerve function, what produced it? What is the mechanism which has become disordered and how, in turn, did this come about?

As we know, nerve tissue is a very specialized type of tissue designed above all else to transmit and receive electrical-type signals. In the voluntary muscular system, there are at all times a constant succession of impulses being transmitted from the brain via the central nervous system and finally arriving at the muscles in such a way as to produce a level of activity in the muscles. This level of activity may be nothing more than rest, which we might call "relaxation"; or it might be up to the extreme end of contraction such as might be required to lift a heavy weight.

These differing levels of activity of muscles—and even

relaxation is activity—require differing levels and balances of nerve messages to be transmitted to the muscles. The balance of these electrical impulses will again vary, but it is clear that the absence of a relaxed state of the muscles is in some way related to disturbance in the rhythmic movement of the brain, which itself is brought about by the inability of the cranial bones to move fully and freely as part of the totality of the cranial rhythmic movement.

The sequence of events might be listed as follows.

Birth Trauma = Cranial Bone Misalignment

Cranial Bone Misalignment = Dysfunction of Motion (Motility) of Brain

Motility Dysfunction of Brain = Disturbance to Nerve Transmission

Nerve Transmission Disturbance = Overcontraction of Voluntary Muscles

The above example of functional disturbance in the body's mechanism refers to what is, in practice, a widespread condition which applies to many, if not most, people. The difference is only in degree.

Further, a similar mechanism exists at the involuntary level of muscles, disturbance to which frequently results in an overcontracted state of the major organs and blood vessels. Moreover, at the level of the involuntary *function* of the body, it is also possible to have an overrelaxed state of structures and tissue. This will also be governed by factors associated with the balance and functioning of that part of the nervous system associated with these areas of function. Either way, overcontracted or overrelaxed, we have dysfunction and abnormality originating at the nerve level which is in turn determined by the efficiency or otherwise at the cranial level.

Nor, we must remember, can we in any way completely separate these two areas of nerve disturbance. If, for example, we have a group of overcontracted muscles at the voluntary level, such a situation is also likely to be influenced by disturbances at the involuntary level. Let's put some flesh on this, if you will pardon the pun.

Suppose there were a heavily contracted group of muscles giving considerable pain and discomfort in the area of the low back. On the premise which I am setting out, the basic cause of such a condition would be nerve disturbance originating within the cranium and having its effects a long way from the cranium. Concomitant with this disturbance of voluntary muscles, it is quite possible—and indeed probable—that at the involuntary level of activity there would be overcontraction of the blood vessels supplying the voluntary muscles. The ensuing narrowing of the blood vessels would then effectively result in a reduced blood supply and therefore reduced nutrition to the voluntary muscles. It therefore becomes a total and interdependent disorder and underlines the need for a holistic understanding of the mechanisms concerned.

It will be noted that, in the case of both the voluntary and involuntary levels of disorder, the origin in both cases is with the dysfunction of the nervous system arising because of disturbances with the cranial mechanism. In Figure 12 the two levels of nerve function can be seen. Nerve A is the one concerned with activating the muscle—telling it what to do— and results in varying degrees of contraction and relaxation to do so. Because of cranial dysfunction, however, there is every probability that there will have been an inherent degree of overcontraction of the muscle to begin with. Nerve B, on the other hand, is concerned with the control of the blood vessels and therefore blood supply and nutrition to the muscle. This is an involuntary function with which we are not consciously concerned, but which will commonly result in a contracting and narrowing process of the blood vessels, as we have seen. And although both functions are separate in one

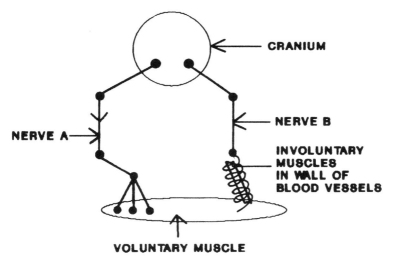

Fig. 12. Nerve Control of Voluntary and Involuntary Muscles

sense, they are both very much influenced by cranial balance, and dysfunction on both levels will exist side by side.

The foregoing examples of differing areas of function, or physiology, give some insight into the essential requirement of the nervous system in order to make virtually every function of the body take place. Without neurological activity, the muscles of the heart do not pump (contract and expand); the circulatory system, which is vital in order to carry the blood supply with all its nutrition for local tissue health, will fail to function effectively; the vital organs, such as kidneys and liver, will be unable to carry out their primal tasks; the glands such as the pituitary, thyroid, and adrenals will not function efficiently. And in the degree to which there is nerve disturbance to any of the functions carried out by any of these organs or systems, so will there be an equivalent degree of organ or system dysfunction. But if there is dysfunction, how come we often *appear* to be functioning in a normal way?

Chapter 11
Disease Causation

The word *disorder* is defined in Dorland's *Medical Dictionary* as "a derangement or abnormality of function."

The word *illness* is defined as "a condition marked by pronounced deviation from the normal healthy state."

The word *disease* is defined as "a definite morbid process having a characteristic train of symptoms."

If a person were suffering from a *disorder*, we would be referring to someone who exhibited clear and unmistakable symptoms that there had been a breakdown in bodily function. We would here include those suffering from NMS types of disturbances such as pain and restriction of the musculature—low back, shoulder, neck, and so on. It would include conditions such as painful menstruation, and it would probably refer to other common abnormalities such as constipation, episodes of nausea or diarrhea, or perhaps long- or short-sightedness. None of these conditions is thought of as being any more than an acceptable deviation from normality of some aspect of bodily function. We do not think of any of these, or similar, conditions as being an illness or disease. Functional disorders are nevertheless common. They may be recurring, with intervening periods of freedom from symptoms; and they may also be so low grade as to be unobtrusive into our consciousness. Thus the very occasional and mild tingling sensation in the little finger is virtually dismissed; a veritable normal abnormality! So, too, would those irritating little herpes, or cold sores, which keep recurring on the lip; or the very inconvenient tummy upset that occurs when a certain item of food is taken. These are not illnesses and certainly not diseases; indeed, are they even disorders? Surely these are, well, normal?

Going up the scale—of downward deterioration, that is—we then encounter the *illnesses* which, by definition, are marked *by pronounced deviation* from normal; and the *diseases* which are defined as having a *definite morbid process*. These two categories are often indistinguishable one from the other but, in general, we tend to consider the more serious or chronic or life-threatening conditions as *diseases* and the less serious ones as *illnesses*. In many ways the differences are academic, but we tend to think of the usually-encountered-by-children-type conditions such as measles, mumps, chicken pox, and whooping cough as being illnesses, not diseases. Such illnesses are of an acute nature, are usually self-correcting, and the symptoms clear in a short time. The same would apply to conditions such as influenza and glandular fever.

While the terms *illness* and *disease* are often interchangeable, we find that *disease* is usually the one to carry the heavier overtones of seriousness. Thus, we will think of conditions such as chronic fatigue syndrome (CFS) or diverticulitis of a low grade as being illnesses rather than diseases, whereas we will think of rheumatoid arthritis, multiple sclerosis, or cancer as being diseases. Whether one even considers a condition to be an illness or disease is often a matter of mere subjective, and often unwitting, decision by the patient or his or her relatives. The medical name of the condition then becomes the determining factor, so that in the early stages of, say, cancer the patient will be described as "ill" and in the later stages as "having cancer"; that is, a specific disease. On the other hand a not immediately life-threatening condition of difficult breathing might be described by its name from the outset: He has emphysema!

But whether a person has a *disorder*, an *illness*, or a *disease* is really of little consequence, providing our attention is not unduly distracted by medical nomenclature which, in general, is no more than a convenient way of describing a particular group of symptoms, the more common ones often being easily recognizable by the laity. What really matters is the need to have some understanding about the basic underlying causative mechanisms within the body which have finally resulted in its producing this, that, or the other group of symptoms which we call *disorder A, illness B,* or *disease C.*

The causes of disease have been the subject of considerable speculation by various cultures over thousands of years. The theories range from the pleasure or displeasure of the gods through astrological influences, through congestions of the body's humors or fluids, through imbalances to the body's energy flows (the yin and yang), up to one of today's favorites already referred to, the virus. Each theory has in turn produced a new set of therapeutic procedures, whether they be incantations, leeches, or drugs. Many have been found to be seriously wanting.

My own view about disease causation, and which I hope will be found to be at least less seriously wanting, is based first on the proposition that the organism, in totality, is potentially a balanced, living, and vital complex and that any departure from this state represents disorder of one kind or another.

At the center of this balanced state, I believe, lies what I have described as the Unit of Function, which constitutes the brain, the cranium, the spinal cord, all the vertebrae, and the dura. Disturbances to this unit, as we have seen with Henry, are all too common, indeed perhaps inescapable. These disturbances occur at or before birth. For an understanding of the disorder/disease-causing mechanisms, it becomes necessary to look at two levels of causation. These are referred to as (a) the underlying or primary or fundamental or *predisposing* cause and (b) the trigger or activating or *precipitating* cause.

These two areas of causation are essentially distinct and separate one from the other and have to be considered as such in order to understand the totality of the two together in the disorder/disease-forming processes.

Predisposing

To be predisposed is to be liable to, or subject to, the onset of a series of events or consequences. In this case it is being suggested that there are predisposing matters in relation to the health of the organism which render it liable to the onset of disorder or disease. In other words, there is an inbuilt weakness or weaknesses which must be taken into account in the disease-causation processes. So what are they and to what extent are they of significance?

From the preceeding pages, it will be understood that the level of activity, or function, of the organism should take place at a theoretically optimum level but that, in practice, such a degree of functional efficiency rarely, if ever, takes place.

Central to this rather sorry, and surprising, state of affairs is my belief that the birthing process, however apparently normal, results in a degree of distortion and warping of the bones of the head which are not fully corrected during the natural process of birth for reasons which we do not yet fully understand. As already noted, there are also difficulties with infants born from cesarean section, but usually of a different nature. In these cases the failure to pass through the birth canal prevents an essential influence on the shape of the cranium taking place.

The misalignment of the cranial bones then, in turn, causes disturbance to the rhythm and flow of the involuntary mechanism of the Unit of Function which includes, of course, the entire nervous system of the body. So we have to try to understand what happens to such things as nerve function as a result of the underlying disturbance within the system to the overall rhythmic activity of the Unit of Function.

It will be remembered that the specialized nature and structure of muscle is that it should expand and contract like a piece of elastic. This is the particular characteristic of muscle. Functionally, it will be in anything between its fully resting state on the one hand and its fully activated, or contracted, state on the other.

In the case of the voluntary muscles, the level of tension, or contraction, will be determined by the message received by the muscles from the nerve supply, including the option to do nothing; that is, to be in a fully rested or relaxed state. If, however, these muscles are not able to achieve the state of full relaxation when they ought to be able to do so, the fault must rest with the neurological control of those muscles—which takes us back to our Unit of Function. I have endeavored to show that neurological function determines the degree of muscular contraction, or tension, not only in the activated state but also in the resting state; and it is in this latter state that the problems begin.

The result of cranial bone abnormalities is to alter neurological function, one of the results of which appears to be to alter the balance of nerve impulses to the muscular tissue in such a way as to inhibit the muscle fibers from being able to assume a fully rested or relaxed state. There is therefore in practice an element of built-in tension in the muscles which ought not to be present. Such preexisting tension will be the precursor, the *predisposing* factor in any particular group of muscles, when activated, going into a further degree of contraction or spasm, giving rise to a painful reaction.

The predisposition, therefore, already exists in the muscular tissue. It is the erstwhile, silent, and insidious phenomenon which is there without our necessarily having any awareness of it. It prepares the ground for the body to react at a later stage. It is the hitherto unrecognized and primary dysfunction within the system. It is symptomless . . . until! If it did not exist—that is, if the muscular tissue were able to assume a fully released and relaxed state—there would not then be a predisposing weakness in the system; the muscles would not be primed and it would be quite impossible for them to react in the ways they do to produce such a variety of painful conditions.

Similar principles apply to the involuntary muscular system, the muscular groups which are part of the complexity of organs, glands, and systems which together sustain the life processes. In this are included the blood vessels, the kidneys, the heart, liver, gallbladder, intestines, lungs, pancreas, spleen, and so much else besides. The level of function of these organs and systems is largely controlled by a section of the nervous system called the "autonomic"; and in a fashion similar to that of the voluntary muscular system, one of the effects of disturbance to the balance of signals being transmitted over the nerve pathways can be to produce a preexisting degree of contraction of the associated involuntary muscles.

In such circumstances where involuntary muscles are unable to assume a fully relaxed state, there are major implications for both the level of health of the local tissue concerned and for the efficient functioning of the organs and systems concerned. If we look for a moment at one aspect of such a situation, it will give some insight into the potential repercussions. All cells must have nutrition in order to be healthy and there must also, of course, be adequate and free drainage to carry off the waste products. The main source of nutrition is from the blood carried as it is through the blood vessels. The heart, for example, not only does the pumping and supplying of blood for transportation throughout the body, but it must itself also have blood supplied to its own tissue via its own set of blood vessels. The same principle of blood supply requirements apply to all the other organs and systems.

If, therefore, there is a primary and permanent degree of contraction of the circular (involuntary) muscles of the blood vessels concerned, then the blood vessel is compressed. As noted previously, it follows that if the tube is compressed so then will the volume of liquid—in this case, blood—be reduced. If the volume of blood is reduced—since blood carries, above all else, the essential nutrients for cellular health—then the level of nutrition to the cells being supplied by those blood vessels is also reduced.

When a heart attack finally occurs, the blame is normally laid squarely at the door of smoking or high cholesterol. In fact these are *precipitating* causes. At a predisposing level, the muscular walls of the coronary arteries are contracted (compressed) with a resultant reduction of local nutrition (blood) and disturbance of drainage: all the stuff to react to the harmful effects of smoking, fatty foods, or just plain stress. Had not the *predisposing* disturbance existed in the first place, then the heart attack would not have happened. I develop this argument in detail in Chapter 12.

These two illustrations about the effects of the inability of the nervous system to function within its normal range because of restrictions and distortions at the cranial level, and the consequential dysfunction at the voluntary and involuntary muscular level, are by no means the only effects of cranial/neural dysfunction. Primary or predisposing contractions of the two muscular systems will frequently be present at the same time, but not necessarily with symptoms, of course.

There are also other areas of dysfunction of a predisposing nature resulting from unbalanced and disturbed neurology. This would include, for example, the ability of organs to function fully and efficiently to perform the tasks for which they were designed. Such matters would clearly be important to the overall health of the organism whose ability to function is compromised from the outset. The organism is therefore weakened from the outset. From this weakness will stem the potential for other consequences to take place. The organism is primed, or *predisposed*, to react to other events or influences of an adverse or threatening nature.

It is in this area of predisposed causation that I believe lies a hitherto unrecognized and vital key to arriving at an understanding of the disorder/diseases processes of a wide range of health problems. After all, if there is an established weakness anywhere in any system to begin with, that system is very much more likely to break down from other stresses. If the gut in the tennis racket is of poor quality, then it will start to fray and break more readily when subjected to the additional strain of play. Whilst the strains to which the racket will be subjected from play will vary from day to day, from match to match the underlying strengths and weaknesses of construction and materials will count for far more in the extent to which failure will occur than in the stresses of play. Similarly with the human organism, the *predisposing* strengths and weaknesses of the central controlling and balancing mechanism, the Unit of Function, will count for much more than the secondary, or precipitating, stress factors.

Chapter 12
Causation: Predisposing

The other side of the equation of disorder/disease causation might simply be put as being the trigger, or *precipitating*, causes. If the organism is primed, weakened, or *predisposed*, then it is ripe to be triggered into a response or reaction as a result of other harmful agents, forces, or influences being brought to bear on the system. It is often at this time that symptoms of one kind will arise in a specific and identifiable way; and, for this reason, it is commonly found that at this confluence of causative influences, the *predisposing* and the *precipitating*, the person seeks a remedy to free him or her from the symptoms. A few examples will help to explain this.

John: Low Back Disorder

John has suffered from intermittent low back pain. He is now thirty-two years old and has been troubled for some ten years. The intensity of the pain has been variable, but he has had three or four acute flare-ups necessitating bed rest and hospitalization. John identified the initial cause of his disorder as going back to an incident when he carried a television set from one room to another. He felt a severe pain at the time in his low back area. Following this, he has had constant trouble in varying degree, the pain often being set off by even the simplest of movements.

Now John, like the rest of us, had his preexisting contractions of muscle groups in the low back area long before he ever lifted the television set. The muscles were already primed. But along with the long-standing contractions of the muscles involved will have been other subtle changes in the nutrition and biochemistry of the muscular tissue.

Because of the disturbance to nerve pathways generally, the blood supply to the muscles will also have been reduced, thus depriving the cells of the muscles of some element of their nutrients. And, alongside this, the predisposing tensions of the muscles will have resulted in pressure on the veins which carry away the normal waste products of metabolism, with the result that potentially irritating metabolic waste products accumulate in the muscles. With reduced blood supply and, therefore, nutrition *to* the muscle cells and impedance to the flow of waste products *from* the cells, we then have all the potential for those cells to become hyperirritable and to react to other stresses or influences introduced into the area—from, say, a lift of a saucepan, a stretch to lift up the baby, or something equally simple.

In the mind of John, the significant—and causative—events were the first episode when he lifted the television set and, to a lesser extent, the simple trigger movements which produced other flare-ups over the years. And this is all very understandable when, so far as he was concerned, he was perfectly all right before he lifted that cursed television set.

Any therapy which seeks to restore health to the individual in this, or indeed any, case must aim at the resolution of the *predisposing* cause which is at the cranial level. Any other relief, however welcome, will continue to leave the *predisposing* factors intact, with all the resultant disturbances to local blood supply, nutrition, and drainage, and its potential for recurrence sooner or later. Whereas clearance of the *predisposing* cause will have not only an immediate effect on the painful muscular tensions, but also on the underlying disturbed biochemistry of the tissue, including any inflammation which is often present.

The type of disorder from which John suffered is widespread in the community and is probably the most common single type of breakdown presented in the offices of most physicians. This, I believe, is because the *predisposing* and neurological aspects of causation are only poorly understood, if at all.

Sarah: Colitis

Sarah, aged twenty-two, suffered from colitis, which is essentially an inflammatory disease of the lower bowel, or colon. She experienced severe abdominal cramps which were usually accompanied by bouts of diarrhea and sometimes bleeding. These acute episodes of diarrhea could occur anywhere between three and eight times per day and had resulted in significant weight loss, partially because of the loss of body fluids.

The condition arose suddenly about thirteen months earlier, some weeks following the death of her brother in a road traffic accident. This emotional factor she considered to be the cause. Drug therapy was only of marginal help, and she had been advised of the early likelihood of surgical removal of part of the colon—all a very distressing prospect and prognosis for a twenty-two-year-old woman.

Perhaps the most significant characteristic of colitis is the presence of inflammation in the bowel. The conventional medical view of inflammation is that it is primarily of bacterial origin and hence therapeutic procedures follow accordingly. But inflammation of any tissue has to be looked at from the point of view that it is an abnormality, a departure from normal, of the characteristics of an area of tissue of normal cellular structure.

The medium, or environment, in which any cell exists must be such as to provide that cell with its basic needs. These may be simply thought of as (a) nutrition to supply the essential health-building materials for the cell and (b) elimination to carry away the waste products of cellular activity. If one or both of these requirements are not being fulfilled in part or in whole then the potential for trouble will exist. The change from normal cellular characteristics to abnormal varies in differing groups of tissue as will be the type of tissue change—inflammation, ulcers, abscesses, tumors, and so on. The lower bowel has a high degree of susceptibility to change, given certain circumstances, from normal to one of inflammation; and it is also recognized to have the susceptibility to change to a malignant condition, again given the right circumstances.

With colitis, therefore, we have to look for changes in the environment of the cells, once again on the two levels of causation, *predisposing* and *precipitating*. The predisposing weakness will have been present long before the onset of symptoms and will have resulted in an underlying disturbance to both the tensions of the involuntary muscular walls of the colon and to the muscular walls of the local blood vessels and, therefore, to the blood supply itself to the essential tissue of the colon. Impedance to drainage of the blood from these parts will also have been present because of the involuntary muscular tensions.

At the *precipitating*, or trigger level, we then have in this case the superimposed or additional contracting factor arising from psychological stress and upset. The resultant additional contraction, probably coupled by other chemical changes from the emotional disturbance throughout the organism, will have finally highlighted the already existing area of weakness. And so there now arises a complex of symptoms which are designated as colitis.

But would the colitis symptoms have arisen following the emotional stress, *had there not already been a preexisting weakness?* I think not. And that weakness will assuredly have been within our understanding of the *predisposing* cause of dysfunction of the organism, to which it is again essential to turn our attention. In Sarah's case she also suffered from low-grade pain in the low back area and had done so for some time before the onset of the colitis. These two areas of disorder—the colitis on the one hand and the low back pain on the other—will too readily be considered as being separate issues requiring different specializations of treatment. The two so-called disorders, however, are both differing aspects of the one causative mechanism. The fact that the symptoms are quite different and in different areas is of no real consequence, and to look upon the totality of that patient in such a fragmented way is to confuse a proper understanding of the disorders. But such things are commonplace.

Bryan: Angina

Bryan is a forty-seven-year-old farmer who suffered from angina. His main symptoms were a feeling of tightness and restriction in the chest which worsened markedly with very little exertion. These symptoms followed his first heart attack three years before, which was severe; and there have been two others since of moderate severity. He was listed for bypass surgery at the time of his first presentation. Bryan's first heart attack happened without any previous warning, as is often the case. It arose through the night and wakened him from his sleep.

The heart is, of course, one of the vital organs and is

largely muscular tissue required to carry out its specialized function of pumping blood throughout the body. And, like all other tissue, it, too, also has to have some of that blood redirected back to itself in order to provide its own nutrition, oxygen, and so on. The problem in angina lies in this transportation of blood back to supply the heart.

The inherent weakness—the predisposing factor—in this case has resulted in the muscular walls of the arteries which supply blood to the heart muscle—the coronary arteries—being contracted and unable to assume the fully relaxed state. Hence we then have the now familiar situation of the narrowed tube through which less fluid—blood—may pass in order to allow the heart muscle to fulfill its normal level of function, which is the continuous working of pumping. If, then, a greater demand is placed on the heart to supply blood to other areas of the body, as from increased exertion, then the heart muscle itself demands more blood, and therefore oxygen, to allow it to fulfill that need. But because of the underlying narrowing processes of the coronary arteries, the additional blood cannot be made available to the pump; and the stress on the heart muscle results in the classic tightening symptoms of the chest, throat, and left arm which we associate with angina. There are often found deposits of fatty materials in the walls of the coronary arteries of patients suffering from angina; and this phenomenon is attributed generally to dietary habits, particularly the intake of foods rich in saturated fats, such as butter, cream, dairy-based products, fatty meats, and similar products. Whilst it is true that the type of food ingested will play *some* part in the fatty deposition processes of the circulatory vessels generally, I believe that such buildups in the coronary arteries arise, in the first instance, because of the *predisposing* contraction of these tissues arising from cranial and related neurological dysfunction (Fig. 13).

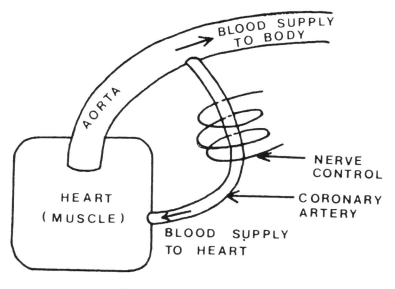

Fig. 13. Blood Supply to Heart

The mechanism of coronary attacks is closely related to that of the occurrence of angina, insofar as there is a preexisting level of tension of the involuntary muscles of the coronary walls—again without symptoms—and because of disturbances to local blood supply to the walls of the arteries themselves, the potential level of irritability of the muscular walls increases, thus providing the mechanism for spasm of the muscular walls to develop. The blood supply to the heart muscles is then severely disrupted or blocked off and results in a coronary episode.

A coronary episode, arising from spasm of the muscles of the coronary arteries, can have probably two secondary but important *precipitating* factors. The first of these is that the level of potential irritation of the muscular walls of the arteries can be significantly increased by a diet which is highly acid forming, including what we call "junk foods."

The second is that, within the context of our Unit of Function, we know that the stresses in the body can be extensive and general because they are often symptomless. In the case of the coronary disorders, the nerve supply is always from the left side of the body and therefore predisposing contraction of tissue on the left side will frequently extend to the voluntary muscles on that same side down to the feet and toes. If, unwittingly, a person with such a pattern of contraction engages in, say, running which in turn will tighten the already contracted muscles in the leg, those leg muscles will contract even further and, through the dura at the base of the spine, will tighten into the cranium. This can have the effect of increasing already existing nerve disturbances—which are even now involving the heart mechanisms—and risk the onset of a coronary episode.

As has been said, no one part of the body exists alone; and here we have a clear case of the potential for the musculature of the leg to affect the heart. We are truly an integrated, interdependent unit whose primary need is balance. And so Bryan required above all else to have the predisposing causation cleared and, by so doing, at a stroke not only cleared the distressing symptoms of the angina but also markedly transformed for the better his potential for a further heart attack.

Finally, let us consider the case of Elizabeth, who suffered a variety of symptoms which might be collectively referred to as female disorders.

Elizabeth: Female Disorders

There can be few, if any, systems in the body which so clearly demonstrate the principle of interdependence than that of the female reproductive system. Elizabeth, aged thirty-nine, suffered from a chronic low back pain which arose after the birth of her first child nineteen years before. She had a history of painful menstruation—dysmenorrhea—most months going back to her teens. But within the past two years or so, menstruation was becoming more irregular in timing; and there was often heavy bleeding. She had been diagnosed as having several uterine fibroids—masses of hard tissue lining the uterus—and, like so many in her age group, had been advised of the need for a hysterectomy. Here we have focal points of an overall disorder showing up as (a) low back pain, (b) abdominal cramps, (c) heavy bleeding, (d) the formation of fibroid masses; and (e) irregular menstruation.

The low back pain, as we have already seen, will be an aspect of the disorder with its predisposing causation manifesting at the level of the voluntary musculature because of its preexisting overcontraction of those muscles. The other four areas of disturbance are more associated with the involuntary areas of function. The dysmenorrhea, which is essentially muscular cramp, arises because of nerve disturbance affecting the muscles at the neck, or cervix, of the uterus. These muscles are so contracted and unable to release sufficiently that there is the resultant cramp when the main muscles in the body of the uterus attempt to expel the blood. The *predisposing* cause is, of course, faulty neurological balance to the uterus essentially related to the cranium; and the *precipitating* cause is nature's requirement during the childbearing years to prepare for the next ovulation process—menstruation.

The heavy bleeding and the formation of fibroids are evidences of the nutritional deterioration which have been ongoing for some time, resulting from the reduction in blood supply to the tissue lining the uterus. This is another example of the effects of the narrowing-of-the-tube factor which has its

81

origin in the neurological imbalance of the muscular walls of the blood vessels, which is again the *predisposing* cause of the tissue changes. The *precipitating* factors in this case are unclear and are probably a combination of stresses, perhaps physical or psychological, or both, over a period of time.

The irregularity of the menstruation process will, as would be expected, highlight the area of function crucial in the whole of the female cycle, which is that of hormonal function and balance. The hormonal activity is at all times an important aspect of the total health requirement, both male and female; but it is arguably even more critical and finely balanced in the female, especially during the reproductive years. At this time any significant deterioration in function will commonly reflect as symptoms of one kind or another.

The female body's hormonal activity is a complex one of changing balances throughout the twenty-eight-day cycle and involves a group of glands called the endocrine glands. These include the pituitary, the thymus, the thyroid, parathyroids, the adrenals, the ovaries, and the pancreas. As part of the overriding intelligence—the Vital Force—of the body, the functional activity of these glands depends upon a constant stream of messages being sent back and forth, thereby allowing each to adjust its level of activity to the overall requirement of the body at any given time.

The level of function of these glands, as one would expect, also falls largely under the control of the nervous system, dysfunction of which is going to have clear repercussions on their performance. Here again we have our *predisposing* causative weakness in the endocrine system which, because of its close association with the female reproductive system, is a primary factor in the disturbances from which the often distraught female suffers.

The foregoing examples are indicative of the primary

role played by the neurological processes in dysfunction of the organism in relation to (a) the *voluntary musculature* with its commonly encountered pain and restrictions; (b) *organ* dysfunction and disease, in the cases referred to, of bowel and heart; and (c) dysfunction of a *system*, in this case the female reproductive system. Here we had an example of the systemic dysfunction side by side with a disorder of the voluntary muscular system, in which the predisposing cause of both lay in the disturbed neurological processes.

It is my belief that without an understanding of the origin of disorder/disease causation, we are not likely to be able to carry constructive therapy very far. The concept of the primacy of the *predisposing* disturbances throughout the body, at every level of function and state of tissue, is essential to the resolution of many, if not most, of the abnormalities from which Mankind suffers. These abnormalities may be dressed up in a plethora of jargon, of symptom complexes, or just mere speculation; but, at the outset, they should be examined and investigated within the context of a *predisposing* causative factor before proceeding to any other level of consideration. For it is here I believe at least most of the answers will be found. *Precipitating* causes of many of our health problems are not to be dismissed, however; but they need to be appreciated for what they are—secondary factors—in order that a more total approach may be brought to bear on any particular problem. It is here proposed to consider some of the precipitating causes of commonly encountered conditions in order to put some perspective on the totality of the situation.

Chapter 13
Causation: Precipitating

There are indeed an almost limitless number of influences, known and unknown, which will have an input for the better or worse into the health levels of each individual. Significantly, perhaps the most commonly recommended and universally accepted option for the better is relaxation which would imply that there is an equally widespread acceptance that its opposite, contraction, is destructive to health. All of which is reminiscent of my contention of the *predisposing* causative factors with their underlying contractive or tension abnormalities.

The survival of the human organism requires that a number of basic requirements be met, and departure from these to a significant or sustained degree will have an adverse effect on the functioning of the organism. For example, we are not likely to survive too long in excessively high or low temperatures, or in an atmosphere of either greatly reduced oxygen supply or increased carbon dioxide. Even this will vary from one group to another, depending upon the degree to which a particular group, tribe, or race has adapted over centuries to conditions which to another group would be intolerable.

Nevertheless, in an increasingly technological world, we find ourselves subjected to many influences which are difficult to quantify in the degree to which they exert a deleterious or even beneficial effect on our general health level. We have nothing but a very unspecific idea of what the use of pesticides, herbicides, and the like are doing to the food we eat, the atmosphere we breathe, and even the water we drink. We have a wealth of *opinion* but very little absolute *fact*. We are told that the increase in emissions of gases into the atmosphere, such as carbon dioxide and methane, is causing changes in the earth's ozone layer; and therefore is ultimately likely to affect our health, if not already doing so. Again, there is much *opinion* but little *fact*. We have the *opinion* that the radiation from our television sets is harmful, but not established *fact*. And so we are often not too sure where to turn to discern fact from fiction, not least of all because of the variety of vested interests involved in the advisory processes.

While, therefore, it is clearly desirable to have as much information as possible about any matters which are potentially threatening to health, it is here proposed to look at some of those factors which by common consent have a causal connection to disorders of the system. There is much research into these factors and development of therapeutic procedures, both simple and complex, to cope with their effects. We consider here what might be *precipitating* causes of a variety of disorders, but exclude what might be called the environmental factors such as those referred to above.

Movement

The act of movement is widely believed to be the cause of much discomfort and pain, which is not surprising when clearly movement X produced pain Y. There is very often a distinct correlation between a particular act and any resultant discomfort; sometimes it is virtually instantaneous.

The most commonly encountered group of symptoms arising from such causes are those previously referred to, involving the voluntary muscles. The underlying causes of these disorders are unquestionably the reasons why the various muscle groups are triggered into a response of accentuated tension. This will then produce symptoms which can be anything from mild discomfort to wholly incapacitating and scarcely bearable pain. Common descriptions of such conditions from patients might be

"I only reached out to put the phone back on the hook when this terrible pain came into my back."

"Just as I stepped out of the shower, this awful pain came out of nowhere."

"I watched the TV for a while and then found I couldn't turn my neck."

It will be noted that each of these episodes arose from normal, nonstressful movement and that, although puzzling in its simplicity of origin to the sufferer, resulted in a level of pain apparently out of all proportion to the mildness of the movement or posture which triggered it. Conventional medicine makes little pretense at understanding the causative factors, and treatment is entirely directly at relieving symptoms. Among the most common therapeutic procedures are bed rest, drugs of the painkiller and antiinflammatory variety, traction, exercises, electrical therapy, and, as a last resort, surgery. In many of these cases the *precipitating* cause can be unbelievably benign and innocuous. So unexpected is the effect that the patient will provide a very detailed description of the events which apparently provoked the pain in the not unreasonable belief that such detail will be helpful to the physician in arriving at a diagnosis of the puzzling condition and, more importantly, prescribing a cure. The role of the *predisposing* weaknesses is not at all understood and hence the resolution of such conditions remains essentially unsatisfactory.

Injuries

In some ways the effects or reactions on the system from injuries are only one step removed from those occurring from simple movement, except that they can be both more severe and more extensive. The circumstances and severity of the injury, such as might occur in a major road traffic accident, will obviously have an important effect here.

Nevertheless, many injuries are relatively minor and the level of trauma sustained can be disconcertingly severe in relation to the nature of the injury. Thus a severe pain in the shoulder, perhaps leading to the frozen shoulder syndrome, might result from a stumble on the steps of the house. The stumble may not have been a particularly awkward one, yet the effect was both painful and persistent. Incidents such as this are in my experience common; but it is difficult to assess their causes, until considered from the point of view of there having been an initial, or *predisposing*, disturbance beforehand.

Sports injuries, broadly speaking, fall into a similar category. In general these types of injury are the lot of younger people, mostly up to about age thirty-five and, of course, apply more to the vigorous types of sport such as football, rugby, squash, racquetball, other types of athletics, and so on.

If we exclude the very severe injuries which can and do occur to athletes, such as a dislocation of the neck of the footballer or the coma of the boxer, the vast majority of injuries have a variety of names such as pulled ligaments, torn cartilages, strained hamstrings, groin strain, tennis elbow, or just plain shoulder injury. In the main these are very un-specific descriptions of the dysfunction and pain, and the feature which is most notable is that they have a habit of becoming recurrent injuries.

It is the strained hamstring which, after rest and perhaps

with intensive massage and ultrasound treatment, finally clears and allows the athlete to resume his sport, only for the whole problem to recur at some later date. The site of the injury will be the same—in this case, the hamstring muscles—and so the process of resolution will be a repeat of the previous time. Such recurring injuries with athletes are commonplace and are the result of the *predisposing* contraction pattern established already within the system. The additional stress superimposed by the sporting activity is the *precipitating* one, which is obviously going to continue all the time that the particular sport is played, hence the frustration and, to the professional, the cost and concern of such a pattern of recurring injuries.

Severe Injuries

Injuries which are severe enough to cause major trauma to the system can arise from a number of sources. In this group would be included fractures, paralysis, and concussion-type injuries. Clearly it would not be surprising if someone who had fallen thirty feet to the ground off a ladder sustained multiple fractures, paralysis, concussion, or, indeed, any number of other injuries. Equally, a similar fate may befall someone involved in a serious road traffic accident. While, even in such severe trauma, the element of *predisposing* weaknesses may have some effect on the extent and severity of the resultant injuries, the major factor here is likely to be the severity of the causes; that is, the *precipitating* factors. But even here we do well to remember that the *predisposing* weaknesses will have some effect on the final outcome but will naturally be difficult to quantify.

In cases where the severity of the trauma is much less, we can surprisingly find ourselves with resultant injuries which can again seem difficult to correlate to the nature of the accident or injury. For example, we have the case of the young fourteen-year-old boy who engages in some horseplay with his friend and falls off a seat in the local public park. Yet he manages to fracture a collarbone. He was not in any way pushed or accidentally trampled on; he just fell.

My own observation over the years with many cases similar to this is that there is frequently evidence of other weaknesses (*predisposing*) both before the injury occurred and in the years after it, *on that same side of the body*, giving rise to the conclusion that, in these cases, the *predisposing* weakness included structural and locally induced nutritional weakness (this will include the contracted blood vessel phenomenon) to the bone tissue itself. But such observations are difficult to prove and for the most must be considered only as matters of probability based on observation.

Totality of Causation

The foregoing examples of the combination of influences required to produce a given effect on the health level might be further understood if we look at it in this way. Let us suppose that there is an arbitrary figure of, say, 100 percent deviation from the norm required in order to produce dysfunction, disturbance, or disease. This figure of 100 percent is the combined total of harmful, or abnormal, forces or influences ranged against the normal working of the organism, which is to say that it is the total of the *predisposing* and *precipitating* forces. The figure of 100 percent may be made up of any breakdown between the two levels of causation. Thus, let us say that in a given case the *predisposing* cause contributes to 60 percent of the symptom onset which, in turn, only then requires a further 40 percent of imposed abnormality from *precipitating* sources for dysfunction to arise.

We can express this as follows.

Case A: Twenty-six year-old footballer with recurring shoulder injury might read

60% *predisposing* cause + 40% *precipitating* cause = symptoms (pain, unable to play, etc.)

On the other hand, if he stops playing, he reduces the level of secondary strain and this might be expressed as

60% *predisposing* + maximum of 20% *precipitating* from normal everyday activities = no symptoms

The *predisposing* influences will in general become more fixed and set as a person ages, as will the biochemical effects on the organism such as from altered local nutrition (blood supply), drainage, and so on. The *predisposing* influences, therefore, become more significant as part of the aging process; but, as a rule, this influence is also in direct proportion to the nature and severity of the cranial injuries—birth. Thus, in Case A, if our young footballer were ten years older, now thirty-six, we might postulate his shoulder injury as follows.

65% *predisposing* cause, requiring only a further 35% from *precipitating* sources to produce symptoms

The *predisposing* factors are the insidious, often silent ones and, in the world of physical stress and exertion, are in reality the cause of underlying weaknesses in the system when the physical exertion *appears* so often to produce the dysfunction. This explains why the prescribed remedy for injury is so often ordinary, everyday rest or, perhaps, some local and peripheral techniques which might accelerate the healing process to some degree; but, all the while the *predisposing* weakness remains untouched.

Allergies

Another common area of disorders is that in which we include a whole range of maladies described as allergic in origin. Allergies are responses on the part of the organism to external influences to which it is particularly sensitive; there is an increased and abnormal susceptibility. The reaction to the allergenic influence, or agent, may range from the mild to the extreme; so that, in some cases, there may be little more than nuisance value discomfort ranging up to the very distressing syndrome where the body seems unable to function normally in anything other than a virtually sterile environment.

The nature and severity of allergies varies considerably from one person to another, even when the allergy-inducing agent is the same or similar. But some of the most common types of allergies are skin eruptions and irritations; discharges of the sensitive mucosal lining of the air passages as in asthma, including asthmatic attacks; reaction of the sensitive nasal and eye tissue, as in hay fever; and irritation of the bowel from particular food substances.

In the allergy type of disorder, much time and effort is spent in trying to discover the nature of the offending, or causative, agent. The hay fever phenomenon is so obviously related to the pollen count in the spring of the year, which also makes it cyclic in its timing, that the diagnosis is usually without doubt; and so the patient is speedily processed to the therapeutic stage. From a practical point of view, it is usually impossible to either remove the offending agent—the pollen—from the atmosphere or to relocate the sufferer in a pollen-free environment; and the usual procedure is to attempt to ameliorate the severity of the symptoms as much as possible. There is no question but that the irritating and trigger substance in these cases is the pollen in the atmosphere. The reason some individuals are susceptible to the influence of the pollen while the majority are not is no doubt the subject of much research but is generally believed to be the result of some factor, perhaps genetic, peculiar to that group of sufferers.

Within our understanding of the causation processes, it is clear that the pollen in this case would be classified within the meaning of the *precipitating* layer of causation. In this case such a perception would be in agreement with the generally accepted medical view. But the underlying and *predisposing* layer of causation has to be looked for within the existing dysfunction of the system which allows a hypersensitivity of the mucous linings to develop, albeit without symptoms, and to react to the presence of a particular exciting cause, the pollen. It is at all times important that the *predisposing* cause be attended to; and, in this case doubly so, since the *precipitating* factors cannot be altered or modified in any way, other than by the use of generally undesirable drugs.

Many skin conditions also come within the classification of allergic conditions and, again, vary enormously in scope and severity from person to person. In this category we have some of the dermatitis-type diseases and some eczemas, all of which are often broken down into subclassifications which describe particular characteristics of each. Such detail is usually of little real value and certainly of no help to the sufferer. In general, we find that the allergic reaction arises either from exciting causes within the system or from irritating influences outside the system.

The main trigger factors within the system are those arising through the food chain. In this respect allergy testing has almost become an industry in its own right, and anyone who has been through such a procedure will almost assuredly have been given a list of substances to which he or she is hypersensitive. These invariably include dairy products such as milk, butter, cream, and cheese. They will also commonly include such varied items as coffee and tomatoes. But those who suffer skin reactions to items ingested in the food chain are often able to list the items to which they, in their own experience, find they are hypersensitive. These can include certain fish (especially shellfish), table salt, and certain fruits such as oranges and strawberries. The list of irritant substances can therefore be contained in foods which are generally believed to be harmful to health, such as coffee, and in foods which are otherwise believed to be healthy, such as fruits. The specific reasons for this are unclear and can only be understood in the general sense of reactions taking place in an abnormal biochemical environment of the body which predisposes it to react in a particular way to certain substances taken into the system.

The list of external substances which trigger off skin reactions is also potentially long. Probably some of the most common of these would be perfumes, lipsticks, skin creams, hair lotions and sprays, diesel oils, washing powders, and even sunlight or certain flowers. In most cases the sufferer of skin reactions is quite clear as to which agent is the culprit and will have often gone to much trouble to isolate the offender by trial and error. In some of these cases, it is possible to alleviate and even apparently cure the skin conditions by merely ensuring that the substance involved is not used any more, though in some cases this can be difficult, especially if the substance is part of the needs of a particular occupation or business; for example, a hairdresser or a horticulturalist. The *predisposition* to such reactions again already exists within the primary and underlying dysfunction of the system which will allow the hypersensitivity to develop. Where the *precipitating* causes are external, it may nonetheless be possible to alter or withdraw these from a person's use or environment sufficiently to allow the symptoms of skin irritation to reduce or clear, even though the predisposing factors remain intact.

Hypersensitivity may manifest itself in many ways, of which the foregoing are some of the more common examples. It may exist, for example, within the alimentary system— stomach, duodenum, intestine, and bowel—and again be related to items in the food chain. Celiac disease is the name of a condition of the bowel in which diarrhea is present and is related to the ingestion of the gluten protein contained in wheat-based products. The condition, which mainly affects children, usually ameliorates by withdrawing all products containing gluten from the diet, which is, of course, to remove the known offending, or *precipitating*, agent.

How often do we hear of the reaction of individuals to the taking of particular drugs which, in turn, were given to help or cure some other disorder in the first place? The fact that there was a condition—or group of symptoms—which justified seeking medical help was itself indicative of the presence of a predisposing disturbance. The nature of this predisposition can then itself become the instrument for the organism to react to the presence of another foreign substance, in this case a drug. The drug then becomes the allergenic agent and, in such circumstances, is then withdrawn usually to be substituted by another. But we are in reality again modifying an allergic reaction by removing a *precipitating* causative agent. The *predisposing* one remains untouched.

Emotional disturbances and shock of either a physical or psychological nature are among the widely varied sources of inducing allergic reactions. It is even possible to be allergic to your mother-in-law! But whether it can be modified or not, it becomes imperative to reach farther back along the line of understanding and to arrive at the *predisposing* issues, the existing dysfunction of the system which allows it to be primed and ready to react to a host of possible irritants.

These conditions can again be illustrated by use of the formula in which it is taken that 100 percent total causative disturbance is required to produce symptoms. In the case of our hay fever sufferer we can express this as follows.

60% predisposing cause + 10% external irritants = *few* or *no symptoms (wintertime)*

whereas

60% predisposing cause + 40% external irritants (pollen) = *symptoms (springtime)*

The need, therefore is to see the precipitating, or trigger, causes for what they are: secondary influences. Or, to put it another way, the imperative is to understand the primacy of the *predisposing* factors in the disease-causation processes.

Chapter 14

The Laterality of Disease

An interesting observation concerning many patients is that a high proportion of them suffer from disorders which relate to structures on either one side of the body or the other; that is, left or right. For example, a patient might present himself with, say, a pain in the right arm, but none in the left arm. Nothing unusual in that, you might say, and such occurrences are ordinary, everyday, matter-of-fact experiences in any medical establishment.

But we know that such a pain in that patient's right arm will have been primarily caused by a *predisposing* factor in the Unit of Function which will have provided the underlying, and hitherto unknown, weakness. All right, it may have been triggered off as a result of lifting that crate of milk, but was he just unlucky that he put more strain on the right arm than on the left? Or was he lucky that the left arm didn't trigger off, too? Or did he put equal strain on both, but it was only the right one which broke down? There is no possible way an answer can be given with certainty to such questions, but . . . there are very decided pointers in these matters.

We have seen how, when the bones of the cranium are in some degree of distortion, the effects of the resultant restrictions in the motion of the bones have a widespread result throughout the system in terms of nerve function, muscular tensions, hormonal function, and so on. The cranial distortions are not necessarily spread equally, as it were, between the left side of the head and the right. They are in practice often very different. The result is that the overall pattern of distortion and disturbance of the cranial bones will produce different patterns on the left side of the head as opposed to the right side. And not only will the patterns on the two sides of the head be different, but that difference in pattern will be reflected throughout the whole of the left and right sides of the Unit of Function, which is to say, the body. There will be a stress pattern on one side quite different from the stress on the other, and this will include a different level of tension or contraction on the one side as compared with the other. These will manifest in the level of susceptibility for symptoms to arise on one side of the body compared to the other. Generally, the more-contracted side at a *predisposing* level will be more susceptible to produce symptoms than the less-contracted side, though this can occasionally be reversed if the difference, from a predisposing point of view, is not great and the *precipitating* factors happen to influence more significantly the less-contracted, or stronger, side. Incidentally, these matters are not in any way connected with whether a person is right- or left-handed or, indeed, right- or left-footed. The strengths and weaknesses, relatively speaking, between the two sides of the body are entirely related to cranial balance, left and right.

A look at a few examples of case histories will help to clarify this important point which is clearly observable in some 70 percent of the population. In the remaining 30 percent, the comparison between the left and right sides is mainly (a) marginal and less well defined, but the restriction and contractions are nevertheless there; (b) more or less equally contracted on both sides, with a similar pattern of distortion throughout both sides; (c) again more or less equally contracted on both sides, but with a very different pattern of stresses throughout each side.

Case 1

Mr. A, thirty-two years old and an accountant, has a painful and bloodshot right eye. He has had this for about ten months and was diagnosed as having conjunctivitis, an inflammatory condition affecting the delicate membrane of the eye and eyelids. Treatment had been symptomatic, consisting mainly of steroid creams and antibiotics.

Further interrogation revealed that this patient also suffered from mild and intermittent discomfort on the right side of the low back area, sometimes extending into the thigh. He had also had a torn cartilage in his right knee removed about ten years before, as a result of a football injury.

And so, we know right away that, first, the eye complaint which brought the patient to seek help in the first place is present in the right eye. The other complaints, one of which continues on and off and for which he did not seek help, are also on the right side of the body. Within the context and understanding of the cranial function and distortion and its determining role in establishing the *predisposing* pattern throughout the body, one is led to the conclusion that Mr. A almost certainly has a higher level of predisposition on the right than on the left side. It is just possible, though, that the left side may have an equal or higher level of *predisposing* weakness but has not yet been subjected to the requisite level of precipitating influences.

Nevertheless, on the side of complaint, the weaknesses are already showing. The picture is one of recurring breakdown on the right side and is one that is likely, if not certain, to continue throughout his lifetime. To the conventional medical mind, there cannot be any connection between this patient's current eye problem and his knee problem ten years before. The orthopedist deals with the cartilage and the eye specialist with the eye: Ne'er the twain shall meet. Why should they? These physicians are trained in symptomatic treatment. The commonality, nevertheless, between Mr. A's eye, knee, and low back problems exists; and each group of symptoms will have had its *predisposing* origin within the cranial level of dysfunction and its overall effect throughout the Unit of Function *on the right side.*

Case 2

Mrs. B, aged fifty-one years and a registered nurse, has chest pains which have been diagnosed as angina. She finds that increasingly the pains develop with relatively little exertion and that everyday walking has become difficult. She is increasingly apprehensive because pains are now occurring in her left arm; and after a series of tests, she has been recommended for a bypass operation of the main arteries to the heart. While it was the deteriorating cardiac disorder which brought this patient to seek help, she also had other symptoms which, to her, were minor by comparison and not worthy of mention until they were elicited during interview. Among these were

(a) the occasional need to have cysts on the left breast aspirated
(b) low-grade diabetes which was controlled by diet
(c) periodic episodes of diarrhea, often accompanied by cramp-type pains in the left abdominal area. She had suffered thirty years before from ulcerative colitis for which surgery—removal of part of the bowel—had been suggested but not carried out.

Already the major symptoms of this patient show up on the left side. The origin of her main complaint, which related to the heart and its main blood vessels, was from the left side of the Unit of Function; the cardiac area is neurologically supplied from the left side. The cysts develop only on the left breast and not the right, and are clear evidence of local disturbance of the mechanisms associated with the health of the breast on one side only.

Diabetes is a disorder of the pancreas in which the secretion of the substance insulin into the blood is disturbed. Insulin is, of course, essential to maintain a constant level of sugar in the blood; and the inability of the pancreas to perform this function becomes a matter for serious concern. The pancreas is neurologically supplied mainly from the left side of the body and disturbances to nerve supply related to this organ will have an effect on pancreatic function.

The other illness of significance referred to by this patient concerned bowel function. The earlier sign of dysfunction here went back some thirty years and was diagnosed as ulcerative colitis; that is, the symptom pattern and investigation fitted that of this particular "disease" which, among other things, is accompanied by high-grade inflammation of the bowel (microorganisms?!) and often serious losses of fluids. It involves the left side of the bowel and usually does not extend to the right. Left-side nerve supply, left-side blood supply and drainage are all part of the *predisposing* mechanisms here; but it clearly comes across that the symptom pattern is one of left-sided stress which will relate to the cranial dysfunction on the left side and its resultant influence throughout the left side of the Unit of Function. There is again a commonality among the heart, the breast, the pancreas, and the bowel symptoms which is not evident in conventional medical thinking.

Case 3

Mr. C, a sixty-eight-year-old retired schoolteacher, suffers from psoriasis, an unpleasant skin disorder which can be of variable intensity. It is characterized by scaly eruptions which appear in patches on any part of the body. The main eruptions in the case of Mr. C were on the scalp, neck, both arms, chest, abdomen, back, hips, and both legs. The patches varied in size, some as small as about half an inch in diameter and others as large as some fifteen inches in length and up to some four inches wide. Apart from the visually disturbing appearance of such a condition, of which many sufferers are self-conscious, it can also result in much discomfort from itching and even bleeding, at times.

The first appearance of the eruptions had been twenty or more years before, and he had been prescribed many local applications in that time and had tried a variety of therapies without success. The patient considered that the onset of the first eruptions more or less coincided with a stressful professional period in his life, but was unsure if this was coincidental.

It transpired that he also suffered from a fairly constant discomfort/pain in the region of his upper back toward the right shoulder blade area and had a persistent pain in the area of the low back on the left side. His history showed that he had had a gallbladder surgically removed about twenty-five years previously as a result of abdominal pains which were diagnosed as being caused by gallstones.

With this patient we have symptoms appearing on both the left and right sides, but the complaint with which he presented himself—the psoriasis—showed skin eruptions more or less equally distributed over the left and right side of the body. In this respect, the psoriasis can be regarded as a generalized or systemic condition whose effects are widespread. The same can be said, for example, of conditions like measles or rheumatoid arthritis, where the disturbance is exhibited throughout the system as a result of what are probably biochemical changes associated with general metabolic activities. The underlying or *predisposing* cause, however, will have arisen primarily on one or other side of the Unit of Function and will have resulted in the systemic changes appearing on a general basis.

The right shoulder blade pain is clear enough and indicates right-sided origin. The gallbladder removal will also indicate right-sided origin, since this organ is also neurologically activated from the right side. In this respect we have two symptom patterns which are clearly of right-sided origin.

On the other hand, we also have the low back pain on the left side, giving us another symptom picture of left-sided disturbance. Two symptoms on the right and one on the left by no means itself is conclusive that the right side is the worst of the two or that the right side is necessarily the one behind the main complaint of this patient. But it has to be said that my own observation of psoriasis complaints points in all cases to disturbed liver function and would appear to indicate some shortfall in one or more of the many and diverse operations performed by this important organ. This may be in some way connected with an inability to elaborate or make available an important biochemical element as part of an often complex chain of activities conducted by the body and which are necessary for health. Whatever the nature of the liver dysfunction, my own provisional conclusions are that it is here that a major part of the psoriasis phenomenon originates; and this is from the right side of the body at a *predisposing* level.

Mr. C also displays a left-sided symptom, but tentative indications are that his right side is the main source of the disorder for which he sought help and that there will again be a relationship between it, his gallbladder removal, and his shoulder blade pain.

In these three case histories, we have seen examples of how a case history will often indicate a pattern of a patient's health over a period of years and, indeed, over a lifetime. This is especially so when we begin to see the picture on the basis of the laterality of disorders over a period of many, or sometimes just a few, years. It also helps to avoid the confusing and often irrelevant appending of names to "diseases," as if each disease was a compartment in itself and was detached from the totality of activity of the rest of the living organism. There is unquestionably a relationship between disorders arising at different periods of time on the same side of the body and, in the case of systemic types of illness such as the psoriasis case, also disorders arising from *predisposing* causes on that same side.

The conventional approach to treatment is to prescribe a particular course of action, be it drugs, surgery, radiation, traction, rest, or whatever else, to deal with the symptoms of each particular episode as they arise: symptomatic treatment. Such an approach is based on the understanding that each symptom complex, as and when it arises, is something quite different from and unrelated to any of the other symptom complexes. What has colitis got to do with angina or diabetes? The answer is a lot, indeed everything; but this can only be seen from a vastly different orientation, an entirely new philosophical—and practical—viewpoint of which no other area of medicine to my knowledge has indicated any awareness.

The therapeutic implications of such an understanding are far-reaching. If we are no longer dealing with symptom complexes on a piecemeal, as-and-when-they-arise basis, we are then dealing with a totality of functional and pathological (tissue change) activities on each side of the body at the one time. On the basis of the *predisposing* causative factors, with their imperative need for change, we are dealing with abnormality involving neurology, organ function, blood supply to and drainage of cells and tissue, hormonal balance, the function of the major systems; in short, every conceivable activity which is part of the health process. We are not dealing with disease "names."

On this basis, Mr. C, our schoolteacher patient, when his first major symptoms came to light—his gallbladder disorder—would have had the right-sided dysfunction in total treated. He would have had the cranial dysfunction corrected and, insofar as this is the determining factor in establishing the level of function of the whole of the Unit of Function on the right side—and the left side, too, for that matter—there would then no longer have been the ongoing basis for further disturbance to develop anywhere on that side. The shoulder blade pain and the psoriasis would no longer have had a predisposing basis on which to develop and would therefore not have arisen.

The history of each individual's health over a lifetime is one of changing symptoms. The primary determining factor will be the degree of abnormality and function arising in relation to cranial balance which, in turn, will set the seal on the functional efficiency throughout the body bilaterally, because of its critical role in determining all other levels of function, such as neurological, hormonal, circulatory, nutritional, electrolytic, cerebrospinal fluid, excretory, and so much else. The appearance of symptoms during that lifetime will be determined also by a range of circumstances which may be haphazard and unpredictable (such as stress both physical and psychological) and predictable (such as age), which will determine some of the body's natural functions and rhythms for that age.

The result is that there is often what *appears* to be a changing picture of symptoms, all of which have the common and primary *predisposing* causative weakness built into the body's workings, in the first instance at the cranial level and, because of this, through the central controlling Unit of Function. Thus, the names of the symptoms change and we are led to believe that we are investigating a series of new problems each time. We are in reality investigating the totality of each patient, guided by the most recent crop of symptoms, but refusing to make the mistake of regarding the symptoms as being the disease "to be attacked."

On this basis we might see a pattern such as the following.

Age 3-5: Little Mary has the usual run of ailments such as measles and chicken pox, both of which were more severe than average.

Age 5: It is noted that she is a hyperactive child.

Age 10: She takes to biting her fingernails.

Age 12: Begins to menstruate; early compared to her contemporaries.

Age 17: Injures her left ankle in a horse-riding accident; slow to heal.

Age 34: Becomes subject to episodes of diarrhea, diagnosed as due to "tummy bugs."

Age 36: Menstruation becomes irregular with increasing loss of blood.

Age 42: Hysterectomy due to fibroid formations in the womb.

Age 50: Severe sciatica in the left leg following several minor episodes of low back pain over a period of twenty-five years.

Age 50: Noises develop in the left ear—tinnitus.

Age 55: Begins to notice tingling sensation in the left arm and fingers.

Age 65: Suffers a coronary episode, survives but develops mild angina symptoms.

Age 73: Suffers fatal coronary episode.

It will be readily apparent that most of Mary's problems developed from a *predisposing* weakness on the left side of her Unit of Function. This is apparent in relation to the ankle injury, the sciatica, the tinnitus, the tingling in the arm, the coronary episodes, and the angina. But some of the other symptoms are also of left-sided origin. The left side of the body might be described as the tension side, and it is frequently found that left-sided disorders of whatever kind are accompanied by an underlying feeling of uneasiness or tension which the sufferer is unable to understand—"I'm just a tense type of person and always have been" or "I'm not tense about anything in particular but just can't shake off this feeling."

Such an underlying state of tension can be observed from childhood: It is the hyperactive child; it is the constant talker; it is the highly sensitive child; it is the nail biter. All these are characteristics of the left-sided syndrome; and although they are not regarded as illnesses or disorders in any real sense when in this childish form, they are nevertheless significant pointers of the potential weaknesses in the years to come. While there are no doubt many influences in determining who and what each of us is and becomes in our lifetimes, it is clear that the effects of the cranial function from birth is one of them. As we have seen, it will greatly set the seal on the level of physiological function and, together with what have been referred to as the *precipitating* influences arising over the years, will have the most profound effect on physical health.

The influences of the laterality of disturbance, however, do also predispose to particular characteristics of personality, such as have been mentioned, arising from disturbance to the left side of the cranium—the bones, this is, and not the brain, of course—with its resultant neurological influences throughout the organism. This will be indicated as much at the psychogenic level as at the physical. After all, the two are only arbitrary divisions of the whole person in any case; and it would be totally irrational to look upon the two areas of "beingness"—the physical and psychological/personality—as being two self-contained, mutually exclusive compartments.

The concept of the functioning of the body—or rather the whole person—on a laterality basis is, I believe, a new one. But it is merely the outcome of the general underlying principles and understandings written about in these pages and explains the basic falsity of the conventional compartmentalization of disease categories, or syndromes. These have to be seen in the context of a deeper level of causation: the *predisposing* weakness with which we are all endowed to a greater or lesser extent from birth and which provides the common thread which enables us to relate what often appear to be totally unconnected disorders one with the other.

On the basis of laterality, it will be obvious from the outset that some disorders result from disturbances on either the left or right side of the Unit of Function; that is, the cranium, to which it is always necessary to return. For example, it would be clear that a pain in the right shoulder originated from disturbance (lesion or subluxation) on the right side; or that the calculus (stone) in the right kidney originated from the right; or that a left-sided sciatica originated from the left side. In order to give further insight into this matter, I have listed below some examples of disease syndromes in relation to their laterality. Some of these are at present tentative conclusions.

Left Side
Angina
Coronary disorders
Hiatus hernia
Gastritis
Gastric ulcer
All-gone, empty feeling soon after eating
Colitis

Simple anemia
Pernicious anemia (tentative)
Hyperthyroidism
Rheumatoid arthritis
Menopausal flushing
Leukemia (tentative)
Diabetes mellitus
Nervous collapse/breakdown
Alcoholism

Right Side
Appendicitis
Duodenal ulcer
Constipation
Nausea
Gallbladder disease
Laryngitis (tentative)
Travel sickness
Hepatitis
Abdominal bloating/distension
Psoriasis (tentative)
Sudden and abnormal loss of energy (tentative); includes
     postviral fatigue syndrome or chronic fatigue syndrome
     (CFS)
Migraine headaches accompanied by vomiting
Depression of unknown origin

Some of the disease syndromes listed above may be indicative of other disorders of the system, and it is always wise for a sufferer to consult a qualified practitioner for advice. The purpose in listing the illnesses and disorders on a lateral basis is to indicate some of the disturbances which can manifest from one side or other and the commonality between them, unilaterally, as they can and do appear and change over a period of years. Thus, there is common ground on the left side between, say, coronary disorders and, say, hiatus hernia or, say, diabetes mellitus. It does not mean that one causes the other or that to develop one of these groups of symptoms necessarily means that another will inevitably arise. But it does indicate that the *predisposing* disturbance on a particular side of the Unit of Function will affect bodily function in ways—symptoms—peculiar to that side; and that it is common, in practice, to find patients who suffer, or have suffered, from more than one of the disorders peculiar to one side or the other. The symptomatic treatment of any of these conditions will result in, at best, nothing more than amelioration of the immediate set of symptoms. It will not have any effect at all on the underlying faulty mechanism of the system and is the reason why it is such common experience to find a changing pattern of symptoms over many years but related to the laterality of the Unit of Function.

Some will, of course, experience symptom patterns indicative of disturbance on both sides. This will vary from those whose symptoms are virtually all one-sided to those whose symptoms appear to be equally divided between both sides. In some 70 percent of patients, my own experience is that symptoms on one side or the other are *primary* and clearly unilateral, indicating the likelihood of that side being the more disturbed—restricted, tighter, misaligned—of the two and therefore more significant in setting and determining the health pattern over that person's lifetime. Some will exhibit virtually no symptoms arising from the other side of the body, but most will exhibit *some* over the years. Yet one or the other side will be the dominant one. The remaining approximate 30 percent of patients will display less marked unilateral disturbance; and symptoms will be more of a bilateral nature, usually indicating marked disturbance on both sides of the Unit of Function and, therefore, cranially.

Chapter 15
Case Histories

If distortion and imbalance of the bones of the head play such an important and primary role in determining the organism's ability to function well, then a look at a few heads might be a worthwhile exercise. And what better one to look at than the one you probably know best: your own? A look in the mirror or, if that is too much for you, a look at your husband, wife, aunts, uncles, or the television screen will provide ample evidence of the gross level of observable abnormalities that exist in all of us. Even without an experienced eye, much of this can be seen in a general way, provided you have some idea of the kind of thing to look for.

First of all, look to see if the head is held vertically. Often, it will be found that, when looking straight ahead, the head will be tilted to one side or the other. When this happens it is the result of muscular imbalances in the neck and shoulder area which are themselves the result of cranial lesions. It is the position of the head to which a person will unwittingly adapt in order to produce the greatest level of comfort and, usually, but not always, indicates that the side to which the head is tilted will be the one with the greater degree of muscular contraction. This can be a pointer in indicating the *major* side in the body; that is, the one in which, in total, is the more contracted. It is, however, not an infallible guide and the opposite can sometimes be the case. But it is a starting point in the observation exercise. In Figure 14 the horizontal and vertical planes are shown for a head held in the normal erect position. The horizontal plane is represented by line A-A and the vertical by line B-B. The dotted lines a-a and b-b represent the horizontal and vertical planes respectively with a tilt of the head to the right.

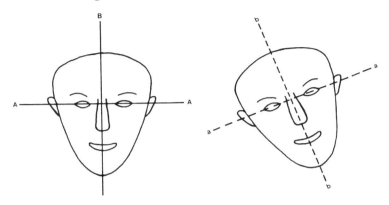

Fig. 14. Vertical and Horizontal Planes

Another common deviation from normal can frequently be seen in relation to the eyes. In this case the horizontal plane may show one eye on a lower level than the other, always allowing, of course, for any tilting of the head that may exist. For example, if the head were tilted to the right and the left eye were lower than the right on the horizontal plane it is possible that the left eye may appear to be higher on superficial observation but will be in reality lower. In a totally symmetrical contoured head, the two eye levels would be the same. Figure 15 shows an example of a head which has the left eye lower than the right on the horizontal plane.

It is also quite possible for one eye to be more receded than the other. To be more accurate, I refer here to the eyes and their immediate surrounding structures up to the forehead and down to the cheekbone, all referred to as the orbits. One orbit may be more receded than the other, indicating a considerable degree of twist, or rotation, of the head in

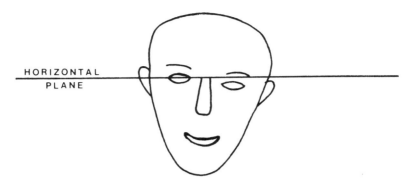

HORIZONTAL
PLANE

Fig. 15. Lower Left Eye

total. This is illustrated in Figure 16, where we view the head from above and see that the right orbit is placed farther back than the left.

A third commonly encountered observation in relation to eyes is that one will look smaller than the other; that is, the amount of eye to be seen in the sockets is not equal. As a rule the "smaller" one is more covered by the lid because the latter has a greater level of flaccidity in the muscles resulting, in turn, from weaker nerve function. There is poorer muscle tone, with the result that one lid is effectively unable to maintain the same level of tone as the other, therefore indicating the possibility of that being the weaker side cranially and, therefore, generally.

Moving away from the eyes, let us consider the ears. These, too, are likely to show a divergence on the horizontal plane and, allowing for head tilt, it is very possible to see the lobe of one ear at a lower level than that of the other. Also, like the eyes, if they are looked at from above the head, one might find one ear farther back on the side of the head than the other on a plane where the two should be exactly opposite one another.

Coming to the nose, one of the most obvious and easily

112

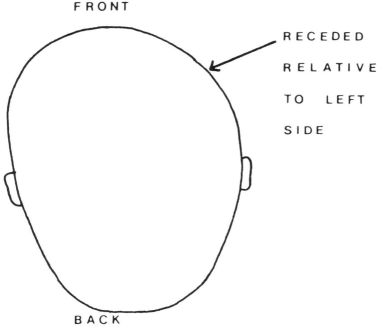

FRONT

RECEDED

RELATIVE

TO   LEFT

SIDE

BACK

Fig. 16. View of Head from Above

observed indications of asymmetry is the nose deviated off the vertical plane. In this area the natural folds of skin which run from the sides of the nose to a point near the edge of the lips will often show differences of depth of crease and in the direction of the folds themselves. It is also possible in some cases to observe differences in such areas as the diameter and shape—round, oval—of the two nostrils, the narrower one usually, but not always, indicating the more contracted side.

And what about the mouth? Teeth are often irregular in a variety of ways, the result of cranial birth malformation and the subsequent determination of the ways the teeth must then grow and develop in order to compensate. There are many ways in which the teeth can be seen to be deviated from a

113

regular pattern, of which probably the most common is to see deviation laterally from the vertical plane. Irregular and overlapping teeth are also common as is a mouth which shows a total rotation to one side or the other of the whole set of teeth, especially the upper. In this case the gap between the two front teeth is significantly off center.

And then, which side of the mouth does a person talk out of? Or what side does he smile from? The cranial dysfunctions, left or right, will often determine which side has the greater degree of muscular disturbance of the facial muscles. The *major* side will often have the more contracted facial muscles and will show up as tightness of movement of the mouth when speaking or smiling. A *major* on the left side, for example, can show as relatively little movement of that side of the mouth with the result that such a person will do most of his or her mouth movements for speech on the right side. Look at your newscasters! Look at the movie stars! Many of these features are evident even to the untrained eye. Remember Bing Crosby? Which side of the mouth did he smile out of and, for that matter, sing out of, too? And which side of the mouth did John Wayne smile and speak out of when directing operations against the stagecoach robbers or the Apaches? I'll leave you to fill in the easy answers.

This difference in balance and level of function, with its relative strengths and weaknesses between the two sides of the body, affects practically all of us and in differing degrees. We are constantly attempting to compensate for the weaker areas in ways that we are totally unaware of every day. When sitting, do you find yourself mostly crossing the right leg over the left or the other way around? When watching television, do you tilt the body in the chair mostly toward one side or the other? When standing talking to someone, do you find yourself shuffling in order to take your weight mainly on one leg or the other? Which side do you sleep on at night? Is it the left or the right? Or do you sleep mostly on your back or face down? Or a mixture of these? All of these are determined by the position in which the body is most comfortable or, putting it another way, the posture which best avoids the greatest degree of discomfort.

The body's own intelligence is constantly at work, without our being necessarily aware of it, in order to allow it to function at its best, given the inherent flaws within. One of the ways in which this will manifest is for us to automatically adjust posture in order to avoid adding to the existing or *predisposing* contractions. Or, again putting it another way, to move into postures which will provide the maximum level of release or relaxation from these contractions. The *predisposing* imbalances, left and right, with their resultant reductions in functional level of the organism are determining our health pattern and our daily lives in more ways than would ever be imagined.

A consideration of a few case histories will indicate both cranial abnormalities and the relationship between them and the health history of the patient. The photographs were taken at the time of each patient's first presentation and before treatment was given.

Patient 1

Our first patient, Mr. A, presented with persistent pain in the low back on the right side, from which he had suffered for some twenty-one years. He had had manipulative and orthopedic treatment at different times but without any success. His right leg was also constantly cold. Mr. A referred to intermittent pain in the area of the right shoulder and also of coldness in the right hand.

It will be seen (Fig. 17) that the head is slightly tilted to the patient's right side with the result that the line of the

115

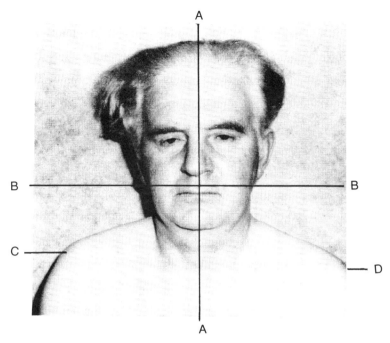

Fig. 17. Mr. A

vertical plane, A-A, is off center. So, too, is the horizontal plane, of course, B-B. But, allowing for the head tilt, it will be seen that the right ear is relatively lower than the left one. The orbit of the right eye is also relatively lower than that on the left side. The muscle groups of the right shoulder, shown at point C, are higher than those of the left, shown at point D, indicating a greater degree of contraction and tension of the muscles on the right side. It will be noted that the distance between the neck and point of the shoulder on the right side is less than that on the left, once again indicating the greater level of contraction of the muscles on the right side. It can be seen also that the folds at the junction of the armpits are higher on the right side than the left, again a consequence of

116

the general "pulling up" tendency of the whole shoulder area from the contracted and tightened muscles in that quadrant.

All of these general observations in relation to asymmetry of the head, indicated by relative positions and relationships of eyes, ears, neck, and shoulders point to a greater level of disturbance with this patient on the right side of the body than the left. These observations and tentative conclusions are confirmed by the symptoms complained of, which are also entirely on the right side of the body.

Patient 2

Mr. B consulted with recurring headaches, sometimes severe, and with nausea, at intervals of one or two per week. The pain always developed at the back of the head on the right side and just above the right eye. He also suffered pain in the area just below the right shoulder blade which was fairly constant. All of these complaints arose following his involvement in a car accident some two years before in which he was aware of having had a slight whiplash injury.

In Figure 18 it will be seen that there is, in this case, little apparent tilt of the head. The rear view of this patient has been shown because it indicates some interesting features more clearly than the front view. The short hair allows us to note that, on the horizontal plane A-A, the right ear is decidedly lower than the left. If, then, we look at the distance between the lobe of each ear and the angle where the neck branches out to the shoulder, that junction on the right side (B) is at a lower level than that on the left (C). So that, although the muscle groups distributing from the neck out to the shoulder actually commence from a lower level at point B, the point of the shoulder on the right side (D) is higher than on the left side (E), suggesting muscular shortening and contraction on

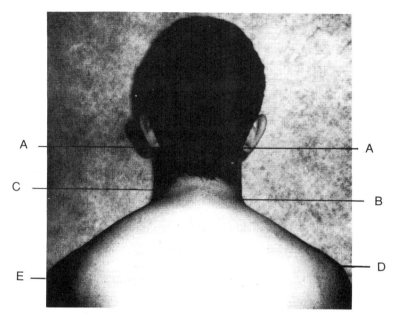

Fig. 18. Mr. B

the right side. It can also be seen that the right ear is further back in the head than the left. All of these factors would lead to preliminary indications of a right sided *major* with this patient which, indeed, are consistent with the symptoms complained of.

Patient 3

This patient, Mr. C, consulted with frequent episodes of severe pain up the left side of his back and extending to the back of the head, also on the left side. They were accompanied by frequent and severe headaches which could last up to five days without remission and recurred at a frequency of about one or twice per week. He also complained of occasional pain in the area of the low back—left sacroiliac joint. Interestingly, he had had severe pain in this same area about four years previously. This had been diagnosed as osteomyelitis and treated with antibiotics on the basis that this disease is of microorganismic origin.

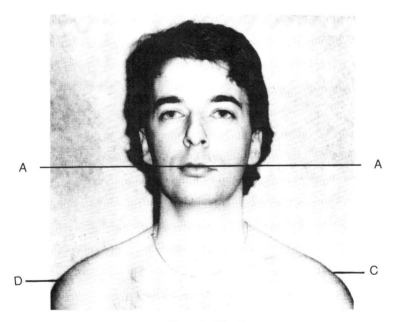

Fig. 19. Mr. C

In Figure 19, it will be seen that the level of the left ear on the horizontal plane A-A is lower than that on the right (the head is slightly tilted to the right); the point of the left shoulder is higher on the left (C) than on the right (D),

119

indicating the probability of greater contraction of the muscle groups on the left shoulder.

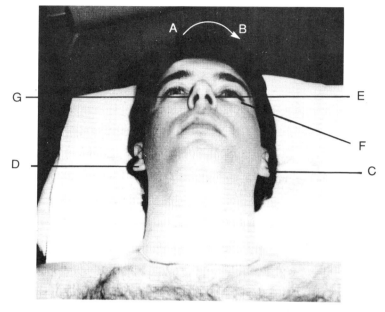

Fig. 20. Mr. C

In Figure 20, we see very clearly the evidence of rotation of the bones of the cranium in a clockwise direction A-B. The left ear (C) is manifestly farther back on the side of the head than the right (D); the left nostril (E) can also be seen to be narrower than the right one (G). The left eye orbit (F) is noticeably farther back than the right one, as part of the rotational process which can be seen to also involve the left side of the forehead. In both the frontal and lower frontal view, the left side of the face shows as being wider than the right side.

The observations here referred to are indications of the

120

likelihood of a left side *major*, which are once again confirmed by the patient's symptoms. The earlier illness of osteomyelitis would be taken to have its *predisposing* origin within the context of the totality of the left side *major* of this patient.

Patient 4

Mrs. D complained of a number of disorders on her first consultation, of which the main ones were pain in the bladder area before and after urination and diagnosed as "interstitial cystitis" bladder weakness which resulted in some degree of incontinence; vaginal thrush intermittently; frequent urge to urinate; generalized low back pain; tension and pain in the neck, both sides; eczema on the inner surfaces of both legs; migraine headaches centering in the area above the right eye which might be accompanied by nausea or flashing lights in the eyes; fluctuation between bouts of constipation and diarrhea; intermittent episodes of palpitation of the heart; large clots of blood during menstruation and severe loss of energy.

This patient's history included a bladder prolapse operation after the birth of her child eight years before; a severe episode of depression which lasted some four months; an outbreak of boils some five years before; and there had been a bladder-stretching operation just four days before she consulted us. All in all, quite a list of symptoms and we had here a patient who had not felt even remotely well for some time. As is usually the case, the patient looked upon her catalog of symptoms as being evidence of disorders which were largely unconnected. What has bladder trouble got to do with skin trouble? What have heart symptoms got to do with diarrhea? What has depression got to do with constipation?

Of all the symptoms referred to only one, the right-sided migraine headaches, specifically identified to one side or the other. Some of the other symptoms, such as depression and constipation, would also tend to confirm as originating on the right side of the Unit of Function and, therefore, right side cranially. Some were unclear as to which side they originated, such as the eczema; and still others pointed to the left side, such as the diarrhea and palpitations.

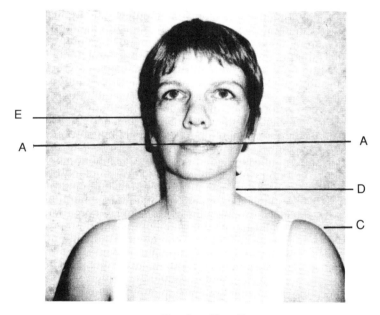

Fig. 21. Mrs. D

In Figure 21, it can be seen that the right eye and right ear are low on the horizontal plane A-A compared to the left. But the left shoulder sits higher at C than on the right, including the muscular line from the shoulder up to where it meets the neck at D. There is also evidence of loss of tone of the muscles of the face on the right side at E. There is not a consistent pattern emerging from these general observations to indicate a *major* on one side or the other, and the symptoms complained of by the patient are indicative of significant dysfunction on both sides. The important point, however, is that, although there is a disparate variety of symptoms, there is nevertheless the commonality of the *predisposing* causation arising at the cranial level, irrespective of the impact of the birth of the patient's child eight years before which precipitated the first of the bladder symptoms.

Patient 5

Mr. E's main complaint had been diagnosed as chronic fatigue syndrome (CFS). He had suffered a weight loss of some twenty-eight pounds within a few months and had little appetite. His energy level had plummeted, and he felt he wanted to sleep all the time. He was also having difficulties with his balance, tending to lurch to the right side. Shortness of breath was constant, and he complained of pain in the area of the lower ribs on the right side.

Mr. E's history was one of having had discharges from both ears and the hearing of the left ear was now reduced. There had also been periods of neck pain, left and right, and an episode of what he described as "echoes in the head." Some twenty years before, he developed a duodenal ulcer which was treated by surgically cutting the nerve supply.

The emaciation in the neck and facial area shows up in Figure 22. The right ear and eye show up as being lower than the left side and the point of the jaw (C) indicates a deviation off center and to the patient's right. There is a considerable difference in the distance between the neck at points D and E and their respective shoulder tips, F and G. D-F is much shorter than E-G, while the junction between neck and

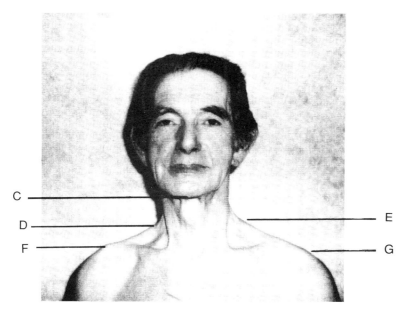

C

D

F

E

G

Fig. 22. Mr. E

shoulder on the left at E is higher on the horizontal plane than at D on the right.

The only symptoms in this patient's history showing up on the left side are the neck pain and the hearing in the left ear, including the discharge episode of both ears. The remainder of the symptoms indicate a right-sided *major*. The loss of weight and appetite point to the possibility of gastric/liver dysfunction, although other possibilities must also be considered; and this would refer to the right side. So also does the duodenal ulcer episode. The balance difficulty relates to the inner ear mechanism on the right side; and, of course, the rib pain is clearly on the right side. The initial pointers are therefore to a right-sided *major*. The main dysfunction here is the chronic fatigue syndrome, which is currently believed by conventional medicine to be of viral origin. But its predisposition lies within the system in the first place; and all sufferers from this complaint, in my experience, have a right-sided disturbance. CFS sufferers also appear to be mainly, though not exclusively as is the case here, female; and one therefore considers the possibility of endocrine (hormonal) dysfunction as being contributory.

Patient 6

Mr. F presented with very clear right-sided symptoms. These were a recurring sty on the lower lid of the right eye; sensitivity and low-grade pain in a circular area of the right temporal, about level with and two inches back from the eye; sensitivity at the base of the skull on the right side; a duodenal ulcer; and a large area of psoriasis on the front of the lower right leg, which developed when he was about ten years old.

The comparison between the two sides of the head and upper trunk (Fig. 23) would, if anything, tend to indicate a left-sided *major* rather than a right, at first superficial sight. The left shoulder is significantly higher and tighter than the right, but the right ear is lower than the left, allowing for the relative lack of flare of both ears from the head. The tone of the small facial muscles on the right side at C indicates weakness by comparison to those on the left.

In all, this patient does not exhibit a clear picture to indicate laterality and reminds us of what can be apparently confusing observations. It must be remembered that a three-dimensional observation will often reveal characteristics which a two-dimensional one, as from a photograph, will not.

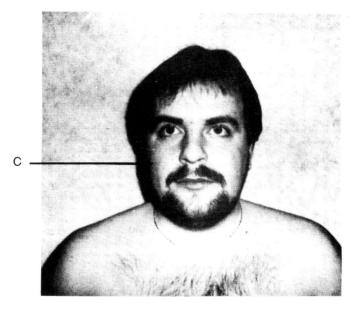

Fig. 23. Mr. F

The main purpose of this exercise, however, is to acquaint the reader with the relationship between cranial distortion and malformations and the widespread effects that these will have, through the Unit of Function, on function throughout each of the two sides of the body. It is necessary to move our thinking away from the concept of treating the symptoms to one of realizing that there are reasons why there are connections between one group of symptoms and another, particularly if they can be related to one side of the body or the other, however far apart they may be geographically in the body. Symptom patterns over a period of years are often continuing manifestations of the fundamental and ongoing disturbance in the system showing up as dysfunctions of the Unit of Function and originating at the cranial level. The understandings and therapeutic procedures for dealing with this are part of Bio Cranial Therapy (B.C.T.).

Chapter 16
Bio Cranial Therapy

There is a widespread assumption, whether explicit or implicit, that improvements in medical knowledge and expertise can only proceed along the same, or similar, lines of research which have dominated medical thinking for the past decades. If this is true, then all we can hope to look forward to is more of the same.

In the preceding pages, I have attempted to describe a new understanding of the genesis of health; and it is hoped the reader will have found it to be at least potentially logical and rational. The mysteries of the living processes, including those of Man, as yet remain matters for philosophical consideration as well as scientific investigation; and it is at once apparent that scientific investigation proceeds apace without any further philosophical pause. Such a state of affairs is regrettable, for science in this field should be the handmaiden of philosophy.

Until relatively recent years, craniopathy has remained in the wings to all but a small number of practitioners within both the osteopathic and chiropractic professions. There is, however, increasing interest in the mechanisms concerned, particularly the involuntary or respiratory motion of the cranial bones and the fixations and abnormal alignment of these bones. For a long time I have believed that within the understanding of craniopathy there were contained the seeds of considerable advances in our knowledge of the total functions of the body and, therefore, in the healing potential contained within it. All that was required was a fuller and more comprehensive understanding of this key element of bodily function, plus the all-important development of the techniques to allow the required objectives to be brought about. The name given to this extension of chiropractic and osteopathy, developed painstakingly over a period of some eleven years, is Bio Cranial Therapy, or B.C.T.

B.C.T. differs from craniopathy in a number of ways of which probably two of the most important are that (a) B.C.T. sees the cranium as being the *essential* determining factor in establishing overall balance and physiological function at a *predisposing* level, whereas craniopathy continues to be seen by different people as offering differing solutions to a more limited range of health problems; and (b) B.C.T. lays down, as part of a philosophical determination, explicit parameters of objectives to be attained *in total* as a necessity for optimum cranial function. This latter point is something of a technical matter which is not appropriate to this book, but is very much a cornerstone of the thinking behind B.C.T.

Man does not just exist. He does not just drift rudderless on the surface of this planet. He *functions* and was designed perfectly to function at level ten on a scale of one to ten. And if Man *functions*, his level of function must be within the control of a basic and primary mechanism. Such a mechanism exists, and this I have called the Unit of Function whose efficiency and ability to operate are above all else determined by factors relating to cranial balance and function.

The Unit of Function is the means whereby the overall and predisposing level of function of so many physiological activities will be determined in the first place. This will include nerve function, muscular tensions (both voluntary and involuntary), level of organ function, circulatory and drainage efficiency, hormonal activity, and cellular function—to name but a few. It will include every function being carried out by every organ. It will include the very essence of what is truly the immune system. It is the totality of function.

The concepts of the *predisposing* and *precipitating* causes of disease, as discussed in this book, are unique to the understanding of B.C.T. While the *precipitating* levels of causation often assume some relative degree of importance and are often identified by lay and professional alike as being *the* cause of a range of disorders, they are, in a B.C.T. context, often of secondary importance. The organism only reacts because of the preexisting causative factors arising cranially and manifesting themselves through the Unit of Function. An understanding of this issue would save much time and suffering in a wide range of disorders.

While B.C.T. is presented as an extension to the disciplines of osteopathy and chiropractic, it is to be understood that the practice of B.C.T. is *not* confined largely or entirely to the treatment of the musculoskeletal types of disorders with which these two schools have become increasingly identified. *The contrary is quite the case.* The reader will have noted in the preceding pages the relationship between disturbed physiology, as manifested by way of an unbalanced Unit of Function, and just about every conceivable bodily dysfunction. It becomes crucial, therefore, to realize that muscular-type disorders are no more or no less a part of dysfunction than the range of so-called medical conditions, whether they be gastritis, asthma, gallstones, cystitis, painful menstruation, tumors, psoriasis, and so much else, with the obvious exception of genetic diseases, of course. This cannot be emphasized enough because, for too long, it has been the increasing practice to separate groups or types of disorders as the prerogative of one set of professionals or the other. But these disorders *all* arise within the *predisposing* mechanism of the Unit of Function and are not just proper to one group or the other. They are different aspects of the total dysfunction of Man.

Bio Cranial Therapy is vitalistic and holistic in concept and application and will, I believe, come to be seen as the foundation stone upon which any conservative and constructive approach to healing must be based. It does not use any of the more forceful high- or low-velocity thrust techniques, but relies on the internal and involuntary movement within the Unit of Function to bring about the required corrections and changes in the body's physiology. It is therefore nontraumatic and eminently suitable even in cases of severe and serious illness, pregnancy, or advanced age.

The results of the application of B.C.T. to a wide range of illnesses at this time are testament to its efficacy, and it is my hope that those looking for an answer to their health problems will find encouragement in the preceding pages that there *is* a rational and logical health philosophy based upon physiology, that we function to the full provided there are not any major irregularities in the works. In short, Bio Cranial Therapy attests that we can be *at ease* within ourselves; that is, free of disease.

Appendix

The teaching of the Bio Cranial System is vested in the Bio Cranial Institute, Inc., whose Chairman is the Discoverer and Developer of the System, and author of this book.

Training in the Bio Cranial System is open to healthcare professionals who have completed a prescribed undergraduate training program.
Further information is available at www.biocranial.com.

Anyone wishing further information, or seeking an accredited Practitioner should check the above website or write to the address below. It will not be possible, however, to engage in personal health inquiries by correspondence.

The Bio Cranial Institute, Inc.,
43-44 Kissena Blvd.,
Flushing, New York 11355

References

Behan, Richard J. *Pain*. New York: D. Appleton & Co., 1926.

British Medical Journal, 1990, pp. 300, 583–586.

Dye, A. August. *The Evolution of Chiropractic*. Published by the author, 1938.

Lyle, T.J. *Physio-Medical Therapeutics, Materia Medica and Pharmacy*. Salem, Ohio: 1896.

Macdonald, George, and W. Hargrave-Wilson. *The Osteopathic Lesion*. London: William Heineman (Medical Books) Ltd., 1935.

Magoun, Harold I. *Osteopathy in the Cranial Field*. Denver, Colo.: Osteopathic Cranial Association and author, 1951.

Pearson, R.B. *Pasteur Plagiarist, Impostor!* Denver, Colo.: Health, Inc., 1942.

Priest, A.W. *Lecture Notes on Physiomedical Therapeutics and Studies in Physiomedicalism*. London: 1969.